"I have known Shawn for a short time as I [...] I have known him for a lifetime through our [...] Huts for Vets weekends. In his book, *The Five Ls,* Shawn masterfully weaves life experiences, humor, tragedy and faith into a must-read guide for those of us in the work of preventing suicide. Shawn, I am so glad to be of Service with you."

—WANDA WRIGHT
Colonel, U.S. Air Force
Director, Arizona Department of Veterans' Service

"In *The Five Ls: A Practical Guide for Helping Loved Ones Heal After Trauma,* author Shawn Banzhaf serves as a trailblazer, lead climber, and guide, as well as Sherpa, charting a course for others while providing much needed sustenance. With humor, pathos, and honesty, Shawn courageously opens his life and heart in a way that provides support and guidance for people in need. He didn't just write this book, he lived it. Shawn draws on his unique combination of skills, education, work experience, military service, and personal characteristics...The *Five Ls* is written for both those who care about someone living with trauma and those dealing with the effects of trauma directly. It is a thoughtful, insightful, and intimate book, at once simple and complex, clear and deep, written with the powerful hope of literally and figuratively saving lives and relationships."

—DENISE ANN BODMAN
Principal Lecturer and Barrett Honors Faculty
T. Denny Sanford School of Social and Family Dynamics, ASU

"Banzhaf's *Five Ls* approach emerges from a place of curiosity, empathy, and compassion. This book is for those who need straightforward solutions for bearing one another's trauma with open-minded love. Whether the framework is directed toward personal or corporate action, I trust the values embodied within Banzhaf's message can be used to guide others toward freedom and wholeheartedness."

—RENEE RONIKA BHATTI-KLUG
Founder and CEO, Culturally Intelligent Training & Consulting LLC

"Once in a while a book is able to weave together theory and practice in such an intricate way that the transitions are barely noticed. *The Five Ls* does just this inviting professionals, lay leaders, family, and those who have experienced trauma into reciprocal spaces of learning and support. Rooted in research but grounded in experience, Shawn offers a book that is highly accessible without being trite or sanitized. His experience in the military is both central to the story and serves as a bridge for other non-military persons. This book offers insight, wisdom, and clear strategies to empower those impacted directly and indirectly by trauma."

— AMY F. JACOBER
PhD, MSW, MDiv

"Shawn Banzhaf, my dear friend and a co-laborer in the trauma informed community movement, created an impactful resource called the *The Five Ls*. He effectively illustrates how to be a helpful companion for those who are suffering and deeply wounded. Shawn's humble but authentic sharing of his life story makes this book both powerful and persuasive. I highly recommend this book to anyone in the field of trauma informed care."

— SANGHOON YOO
Founder of The Faithful City and Arizona Trauma Informed Faith Community

"God is light. We, humankind, men and women alike, have been made in God's image. Trauma accentuates the nature of our human condition. We all need the *Five Ls* – to use them in helping the ones we choose to love and we need them to be used by those who choose to love us. These are tremendously powerful, practical steps we desperately need for healing."

— STEVEN BORDEN
Retired Captain, U.S. Navy
Associate Vice President, Military Programs, National University

The Five Ls

A PRACTICAL GUIDE FOR HELPING LOVED ONES HEAL AFTER TRAUMA

SHAWN BANZHAF

Assisted by
Jamin Andreas Hübner

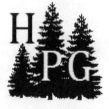

Hills Publishing Group • Rapid City, South Dakota

Hills Publishing Group
Rapid City, South Dakota
www.hillspublishinggroup.com

Printed in the United States of America with chlorine-free, acid-free ink on 55# paper made from 30% post-consumer waste recycled material
Cover photo of Jessica Hübner by Jamin Andreas Hübner, taken north of Avon, South Dakota

ISBN: 978-0-9905943-7-6

Typeset in Palatino Linotype, inspired by Giambattista Palatino (1515-1575), designed by Hermann Zapf (1918-2015) and originally produced by the Stempel foundry (1895-1986) in Frankfurt, Germany.

BISAC Subject Headings:
    FAM055000 FAMILY & RELATIONSHIPS / Military Families
    PSY022040 PSYCHOLOGY / Psychopathology / Post-Traumatic Stress Disorder (PTSD)
    SEL043000 SELF-HELP / Post-Traumatic Stress Disorder (PTSD)

About the Author

Shawn Banzhaf (BA Interdisciplinary Studies; MA Sociology, i.p.) currently serves as the Senior Military Advocate for Arizona State University, a Senior Trainer and Consultant for veteran and military affiliated persons at Culturally Intelligent Training and Consulting LLC, and as a Board Member of First Page in Colorado, an organization that helps the children of veterans with trauma. He formerly served as a Police Sergeant, associate pastor, university campus minister, and is a retired Platoon Sergeant from the U.S. Army National Guard (1990-2012), which included a twelve-month combat tour in support of Operation Iraqi Freedom. Shawn lives with his wife Jodi in the Tempe area and have two adult children and four grandchildren.

Instagram and LinkedIn: shawnbanzhaf
Facebook: shawnbanzhaf1
Email: banzhaf5ls@gmail.com

About the Assistant Author

Jamin Andreas Hübner (BA, MA, MS, ThD) is a Research Fellow for the Center of Faith and Human Flourishing at LCC International University (Lithuania), and a professor in the social sciences at The University of the People (global) and Western Dakota Tech (Rapid City, SD). He formerly served as a Director of Institutional Effectiveness, Department Chair, and Academic Dean in liberal arts higher education. His scholarship is interdisciplinary with research focusing primarily on intersections of religion, gender, economics, and social justice. He lives with Jessica in the (stolen) Black Hills of South Dakota with their two dogs and tarantulas.

CONTENTS

THE FIVE Ls

For Jodi
Who loved, listened, learned, lessened, and led

ACKNOWLEDGEMENTS

I would first like to blame this book on Jamin, without whom this volume would not exist. You may have laughed, but I never anticipated being able to write a book at any scale until Jamin encouraged me to do so. His dedication to the cause of helping people walk through trauma speaks for itself through his everyday life. Thank you Jamin for your support and dedication of this publication. I will forever be indebted to you.

Thank you to all of those whom I had the distinct honor of serving with as part of the military, law enforcement, and the church. As colleagues in the fight for the betterment of society, I hold in high regard the moments in my life that we stood shoulder to shoulder.

Steve Borden, thank you sir, for taking a chance on me as the Chaplain of the Pat Tillman Veteran's Center. And, to Michelle Loposky, for your friendship and your dedication to bring a holistic approach to providing for our student veterans at the Center (but even more for making sure my head doesn't get too big in the work that I am doing). Thanks, Boss Lady.

I would also like to thank Matt Schmidt for encouraging me to write my first LinkedIn article and for telling me I had a knack for telling stories that should be published for others to benefit from.

Thanks to Jamin, Jodi, and others in preparing and contributing to the manuscript, including Jessica Hübner ("Lenny"), for completely revamping chapter three. All mistakes are my own and (quick disclaimer!) I write this work as an independent author; I'm not speaking on behalf of any school, organization, or individual.

I also want to dedicate a few lines to thank my children for their support and for believing that I could somehow embody the superhero in their lives. Zachary (Buddo), thank you for stepping in and being "the man of the house" while I was deployed. I know now that this created in you something I would never have wanted, as you hid away the struggle to never want to bother me with your problems. You are and will always be a better man than me. I am honored to be your dad. To Zach's wife, Nicky, thank you for encouraging my writing and for being the perfect match to our son. Your heart for people is evident and I am excited for your own writing future. You have great things ahead of you.

And to Jenna (Bug). How you were able to maintain the happiness in life even as your father left you at such a young age to go fight in a war — which now seems a very sad reason to leave a 10-year-old daughter at home without her daddy. I see your positivity and it emanates from you. It is truly a gift to the world around you. A better daughter could never be found. I am humbled to be your father. To Jenna's husband, Javaris, thank you for honoring me by taking care of my daughter and being such a wonderful father. You will, I am sure, accomplish great things on your journey in graphic design!

And to my grandkids, I pray that one day the legacy that I leave you will not be one of how tough of a soldier your grandpa was or how much he could bench press (455lbs, oh yeah!) but a legacy of love. That when my name is uttered in passing at your Thanksgiving Day feast many years from now you, will speak of the undying love that I showed you, your parents and your grandma. Remember this quote (and I am sure I am not the first one to pen it but I have claimed it as my own): "There is no such thing as a love crime." In all you do, love well.

And of course, to Jodi, where all words fail, and to whom this entire book is dedicated.

Shawn Banzhaf
Phoenix, Arizona
January, 2021

FOREWORD

Shawn Banzhaf is a rare mix of practical thinking and idealistic action. A man of faith and reverence, Shawn's sensitivity to others is the definition of empathy. This book represents an empathetic union of thought and action toward overcoming stressful life challenges and becoming the best person you can be.

When I first met Shawn in 2018, he was a participant in Huts For Vets, a unique program I created for military veterans in the wilderness of the Rocky Mountains. Together, we hiked mountain trails, shared meals and discussed philosophy in a rustic cabin surrounded by wilderness at 11,000 feet. We found our common bond in striving to humanize the traumas of war incurred through service to a greater good.

This is where Shawn fully revealed his philosophical depth. Not willing to accept failings and faults, either in himself or in the social institutions he serves, Shawn has blazed a trail to our better selves through simple, yet profound, intent. This book is an invitation to becoming more aware of how we interact with each other by advancing five fundamental, yet nuanced, disciplines.

Shawn's approach is uniquely Shawn, in that his innovative mindset has created a methodology that has worked for him and can work for others. Rather than a self-help book, *The Five Ls* provides a platform for social evolution through intentionally beneficial, interpersonal relations.

Rather than paraphrase Shawn's ideas here on love, listening, learning, lessening, and leading, I will let Shawn's writing and thinking stand on their own as a marker of a man who deeply cares and whose heart and soul are represented in every word. Shawn's motive for writing this book is pure: *to advance human relations through selfless care of self and support of others.*

As a member of the Nebraska Army National Guard who faced life-altering combat deployments in Iraq, Shawn gave of himself at a high level of sacrificial service to his country. With this book, Shawn, now armed with the purpose and meaning he has embraced in his life, is giving a deeper part of himself to the still greater service of humanity. This is the path he has blazed to true leadership through ideals and action.

Paul Andersen
Founder and Executive Director
Huts for Vets Wilderness Healing for Veterans

Complications: my claim to fame
And I can't believe there's another
Constantly just another
Can't avoid what I can't control
And I'm losing ground, still I can't stand down
I know, yeah, I know, yeah

I know you stay true when my world is false
Everything around's breaking down to chaos
I always see you when my sight is lost
Everything around's breaking down to chaos
I know you stay true when my world is false
Everything around's breaking down to chaos
I always see you when my sight is lost
Everything around's breaking down to chaos

It's hard to trust anyone again
After all the letdowns I've been through
Haunted by what I've been through
Best to try while I still can breathe
And I'm screaming out, "give me help somehow"
And I know, yeah, I know, yeah...

"Chaos"

MUTEMATH

INTRODUCTION

THE SUICIDE PLAGUE

Traumatized, we find ourselves chained to a past that we feel doomed to forever repeat; like the souls in Dante's *Inferno*. Sometimes…death feels like the only option. Suicide may seem, in desperate moments, to ratify our despair or demonstrate our loyalty to those we've lost.

Twenty US veterans kill themselves everyday.[1]

That's about one every hour. And it seems not to be getting any better.

Graph 3. Unadjusted and Age- and Sex-Adjusted Suicide Rates for Veterans and Non-Veteran Adults (2005–2017)

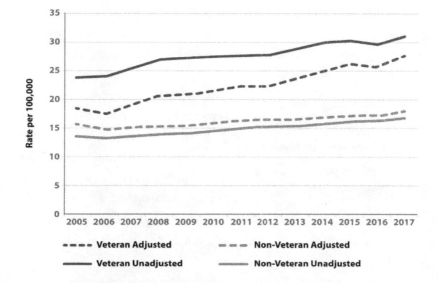

As the same report summarizes:

- The number of veteran suicides exceeded 6,000 each year from 2008 to 2017.
- Among U.S. adults, the average number of suicides per day rose from 86.6 in 2005 to 124.4 in 2017. These numbers included 15.9 Veteran suicides per day in 2005 and 16.8 in 2017.
- In 2017, the suicide rate for veterans was 1.5 times the rate for non-Veteran adults, after adjusting for population differences in age and sex.
- According to stopsoldiersuicide.org, "Since 2006, there has been an 86% increase in suicide rate among 18-to-34 year old male veterans." Furthermore, 39,000 U.S. veterans are homeless on any given day; these variables are certainly related.
- *Far* more U.S. soldiers die of suicide than in combat.

It's statistics like these that leaves me shocked and speechless.[2]

How? Why? What should we do? What can we do?

I hate to start this book on a somber tone, but we have got to come to grips with reality here: the biggest danger for soldiers isn't bombs and bullets on a foreign battlefield; it's something within our own borders—lurking in very our own homes.

"By 2030, the total of veteran suicides will be 23x higher than the number of post-9/11 combat deaths."
(stopsoldiersuicide.org)

There are few things as traumatizing as war. And there are few challenges like engaging in combat for several years and then going back home and trying to live a "normal life." This isn't just "somebody" out there. These are our loved ones—our friends, sons and daughters, husbands and wives, mothers and fathers. It's not a group that's isolated from society.

And as we ask ourselves primitive questions like these, there are some primitive answers that we have to reckon with all the same:

INTRODUCTION

We have to do everything we can to stop killing each other.

We have to do everything we can to stop killing ourselves.

We must end war, and end suicide.

Humans have been on this planet for a really long time, sent people to the moon and split the atom—*and we still haven't figured these two things out.* Oh, I know, "There will always be war." "People will always kill themselves." "So, give up. It's hopeless."

Soldiers don't give up.[3]

So, for this book, I'm going to let the political philosophers, peace activists, and ethicists address the first problem about war and national violence, and I'll focus on the second one instead:

How do we keep people from committing suicide, and reduce the suffering of those with, and affected by, PTSD?

I realize that's a huge, *huge* question. It seems larger than life. It's not something anyone is really prepared to address.

And it certainly wasn't why I left rural Nebraska for the desert metropolis of Phoenix, Arizona…

HOW I GOT HERE

The story begins with what some would describe as "a hint of the miraculous."

As the new associate pastor of a church near the Arizona State University (ASU) campus, I decided that since I had about seven years dealing directly with college students, it was only sensical that I try to make some connections at the university. So, being the typical campus-missionary minded person that I was at that time, I drove to the campus and wandered about this enormous place in search for one of those "divinely appointed" moments. But, as some of you already know, what's always interesting about these kinds of moments is that, when they come, they do not exactly come as anticipated.

Jodi (my wife) and I moved to Phoenix because we had it on our hearts to minister to the needs of international students, and ASU had a huge international student population (over 12,000). Realizing one statistic about their journey here in the United States fueled that fondness: International students that come to study in the U.S. bring gifts for when they're invited into someone's home, but most return to their homeland after four years *with* the gift. Why? Because they simply weren't invited to anyone's home, so there was no one to give it to! The U.S. (evidently) isn't as welcoming to foreigners as some of us imagine. With a background in helping college students, it seemed clear what we should do and why we should leave Nebraska for Arizona.

But our planned journey took an unexpected detour after I actually started visiting the campus. As I wandered around the student union area and went into the lower level to grab some lunch, I noticed a sign on the door that said something about a veteran's center. I felt something tug inside of me and heard a small voice that said, *go in*. I ignored it, actually chalking it up to my apparent weaknesses. I told myself that it was me wanting the safety and security of things that I know well (being a veteran), but I was here for other reasons. Going in that door would mean I was taking an "easy" path.

I walked past the door and sat down with my lunch.

As I was there for a few moments attending to my meal, a young man walked up and asked if he could sit next to me in the open seat. He continued, "I'm a veteran and noticed your backpack and I see you are a veteran, too." I looked down and realized that I did indeed have my "go bag" with my camouflaged name tag on it. We then had a nice conversation about the struggles of coming to the university out of the Army and how he was navigating it.

The next day, I again went back to the university and the student union, by the veteran's center, and the same small voice said, *go in*. I was determined, however, to "stick to my mission" and find international students to strike up a conversation. Lunchtime rolled around and again a young man, a different one this time, walked by. And again, the young man says, "I see that you are a veteran. I am, too. I served in the Navy and just got out." And we talked...as if this was a kind of replay, and as if, well, *as if this is what I was there to do.*

And it got me thinking: what if it was?

A third day, I went back to the same spot, heard the same small voice, got my lunch, but no veterans sat down. So, I thought, *See? I'm not really supposed to go into the veteran's center; I already know my "divine calling."* I finished my lunch and walked out to the commuter shuttle provided by the university. Students were standing around an area waiting, and then I looked over and saw a young man, black cap, formed bill, dark sunglasses, short hairstyle wearing what I knew to be a "go bag" like mine. I said to myself, "OK, there's a veteran." As we filed on the shuttle, both of us afforded others the chance to get on the shuttle first (as is custom to do for civilians in military culture). We were the last two to get on.

And you know what happened, right? There were only two seats left—and they were directly across from one another! So, this time, I said, "So, you must be a veteran?" He replied in the affirmative, and I found out that he recently started school here, had a wife and child, but was struggling with the transition into civilian life just like the other two veterans I spoke to.

Now if you are keeping track, three times I heard this small voice saying to go into the veteran's center, and three times I said "no," and all three times a young student veteran was put in my path so that I basically had to talk with them.

It was time to swallow whatever hesitance I had and just check it out. Whether it was just "coincidence" or not, it was clear enough to me what I was supposed to do.

The next week rolled around and I went to a group meeting of other campus pastors. I had talked to my senior pastor about whom I should speak with in regards to getting connected to the veteran's center, and I wondered if any other ministries on campus had connected with them. Pastor gave me a name, and I decided to speak to him before the meeting. I did so, and then *he* gave me a name and said that this veterans-connected person should actually be at this meeting…*today,* and I should talk to him. This is where things got interesting.

During our roundtable discussions with about 20 or so people, we were discussing all kinds of things. But then, all of the sudden, out of nowhere, this older gentleman literally stands up (and appeared to have some sort of service dog with him), and declares with much enthusiasm that "I think someone should do ministry to our veterans!" If a photo could have been taken of me at that moment, my jaw would be on the floor. I inferred that this must have been the man that I was supposed to talk to—and so I intended to right away after the meeting. However, he left while I was speaking to another campus pastor, so that chance was missed.

...Until I finally did it: I walked into the veteran's center to talk to him. I went up to the front desk and asked the guys working there if I could speak to the director. One of them advised that he wasn't around at the moment but I could leave a message. So, I wrote him a sticky note:

> Dear Sir, I saw you at the meeting today and I would like to talk to you
> about volunteering my time to be the chaplain for this center.
> Shawn Banzhaf [phone] [email]

It wasn't a few hours and I received a phone call from the director. We set up a lunch meeting for the following week. On the day of the meeting, I arrived a bit early. I figured I should probably learn something about him and the center while I had the time. After a quick Google search and some reading, I realized that this guy wasn't the person I had seen at the meeting. He was someone completely different! Now I was really confused (who was the prophet-like figure with the dog?), but it was too late to back out now.

We ended up having a great conversation. He told me that the day I had stopped by the office, he had been pondering a particular idea: adding services to the center that veterans already enjoyed while on active duty. This meant bringing on a chaplain. He continued and told me, "Then I got your sticky note and was assured that God must have heard my prayer and quickly made the call to connect with you." I was never supposed to have even met with this guy! And here it was, an open door, supply and demand instantly fulfilled. I obviously asked him about the other man with the dog and, to my surprise, he had no idea who he was.

This was…weird. So, I went back the next day to the place where we had our campus pastors meeting and began asking people who the man was—the older guy with the dog who proposed a veteran's ministry at the university. They all probably knew him as a longtime attendee and local figure, so this was an easy answer.

No one could tell me who he was. In fact, they assured me that it was the only meeting where they had seen him.[4]

MY WORK, AND YOURS, WITH VETERANS AND THE TRAUMATIZED

So that's the quaint little story that led me to be the volunteer chaplain for the Pat Tillman Veterans Center at Arizona State University.

I spent two years in that capacity and was asked to apply to the position that I currently hold, which is the Senior Military Advocate. I now spend my days helping student veterans (like the three I had spoken to) walk the transition from military life to civilian life, and help them with the struggles they face, coping with the traumas of war and this world. I've learned a lot—a lot about grief, about PTSD (Post-Traumatic Stress Disorder), about family dynamics, and about social change. My graduate studies in sociology here at ASU have also opened my eyes to new dimensions of these challenges and experiences. I continue to learn and evolve as a person, and I'm encouraged by what a difference my time and effort can make in the lives of those who have given up so much.

And if *I* can actually help people struggling with various kinds of traumas, why can't *you*?

So, when the idea for this book came into being, it seemed obvious that it should be written. I can't help everyone. But *all of us together*, across the country, across the globe, can influence the one or two people in our lives in a positive way. The end result would be a dramatic restoration towards human flourishing.

That's my goal—and I do believe we can make it happen.

THIS BOOK

This book is based on a series of talks I've delivered at various venues as part of my work with veterans and others affected by PTSD. So the material in this book is quite "grassroots," even as many of the themes are familiar to many.[5] Most of the books on trauma cited in this book came after I had already wrote it. Jamin (my assistant author, editor, and publisher) felt it was necessary to corroborate with secondary sources to reinforce different aspects, bring awareness to the writings of others, and integrate the ongoing conversation on this subject. Neither of us are really scholars on PTSD, after all. Nevertheless, it is something I personally deal with and help others with on a daily basis, and it's an area that I'm extremely familiar with both from the inside looking out, and the outside looking in.

There's an ocean of books on trauma out there, and each has their own particular angle and perspective. I don't claim to know any more than the specialists, or to reveal some secret magic. But what I do know is what helped me, what has helped others, and (at least in part) why these strategies have worked. That's why the subtitle of this book is "a practical guide for helping loved ones heal after trauma." It's not a book about neuroscience, medicine, or traditional psychology and anthropology, but about the more concrete, interpersonal pragmatics of coping with what is now called "post-traumatic stress disorder."[6] It's about how relationships and relational dynamics provide the scaffolding necessary for restoration—relationships to people, to nature, and to our own selves. No one is an island.

What makes the Five Ls particularly different is that it is primarily designed for partners and allies—for those who are caught up in someone else's PTSD.

But what makes *The Five Ls* particularly different is that it is primarily designed for partners and allies—for those who are caught up in *someone else's* PTSD. The reader I'm talking to in this book is usually the spouse or partner or friend of the one whose relationships and lives changed after the traumatized person came back from war (or whatever events they experienced). I do sometimes speak to the traumatized throughout the book and, in a way, anyone affected by PTSD. Nevertheless, in the end, my approach is simple: "You wanna help people like me and others dealing with PTSD? Here you go: the five Ls that worked for me."

Many may interpret parts of this book as being simplistic and unqualified, while others may find some parts too deep and complex. I unfortunately cannot satisfy everyone. Furthermore, while I trust that my experience, story, and education is

> *In the end, my approach is simple: "You wanna help people like me and others dealing with PTSD? Here you go: five Ls that worked for me."*

adequate for writing a book like this, it remains limited. I can't speak for everyone in every time or place. I know the horrors of war, but other traumas I can't attest to. I come from a religious background in a broadly Protestant-evangelical tradition, so certain references may not make sense to Muslims or Hindus or agnostics or whatever religion you may affiliate with. I'm a white male heterosexual with privileges I don't even understand yet (though one of them is not having my dignity or rights questioned in any U.S. Supreme Court decision). Appealing to Jodi in my own marriage as an example of therapeutic love throughout the book was an honor and something I hope is helpful, but it also has its risks and may even be triggering for some wives of veterans who have sacrificed too much of themselves and need support for their own PTSD. I can only say that (a) my own story may not be your story, but my past and present experience is the only starting point I have; (b) I don't mean to invalidate anyone else's experience by sharing mine, and (c) I want this book to be as accessible as possible, for whoever the audience may be.

And if it helps you at all, it was worth it for both of us. As chapter three will suggest, there is much to learn, and I hope this book is not the end, but the *beginning*, of an important and transformative journey.

THE FIVE Ls IN SUMMARY

How do we effectively help our loved ones who are suffering from trauma? And help not just veterans who are suffering, but *anyone*—like survivors of cancer, sexual assault, or abusive relationships?

That's the question of this book, and it proposes a straightforward, no nonsense approach:

1. We *love* them.
2. We *listen* to them.
3. We *learn* about them and their trauma.
4. We *lessen* the opportunity for further trauma.
5. We continually *lead* them to a less chaotic place on this whole journey.

Love is first and the most important because without putting others ahead of ourselves and being willing to enter into their experience, we can't go anywhere at all. We remain isolated and powerless, like a lightbulb without electricity. This first chapter calls for radical empathy and patience in a world that pushes us in the other direction.

With love in place, all the other Ls can occur. By *listening* to our loved ones, they feel heard, validated, and we become changed ourselves. By *learning* about trauma and their experience, we learn not to take the effects of PTSD personally, learn how to avoid fear, and learn how to ask the right kinds of questions that unfold the layers, heal, and fosters growth in their transformed identity. By *lessening*, we protect our loved ones from being needlessly triggered and anxious. And by *leading*, we can (and will) help our loved ones find order amidst chaos.

Anyone can perform these skills at any time and in any order, though (a) they do overlap, and (b) love is the precondition for all of them.

I've been using the Five Ls for some time now, and can say with confidence that it's effective, and really speaks to people where they're at. I hope you come to find this approach powerful and effective as well.

The Five Ls

Love

Listen

Learn

Lessen

Lead

Compassion is the radicalism of our time.

—DALI LAMA

Friends show their love in times of trouble,

not happiness.

—EURIPIDES

The chance to love and be loved exists no matter where you are.

—OPRAH WINFREY

Love is a movement. Love is a revolution. This is redemption. We don't have to slow back down. We're starting now.

—SWITCHFOOT

Now faith, hope, and love remain—these three things—and the greatest of these is love.

—1 CORINTHIANS 13:13

The only demand of life is the privilege to love all.

—SWAMI CHINMAYANANDA

A life devoid of love is a flower blooming in the wilderness, with nobody to enjoy its fragrance.

—KABIR JI, GAURI RAG

God is love.

—1 JOHN 4:8

1

LOVE

WHAT CAN I DO TO HELP?

One of the most frequently asked questions I come across as I help veterans and others dealing with trauma is this:

"What can I do to help?"

It's a simple and well-known question, but it has several important implications that can easily be overlooked.

First, it shows the heart of the person asking. If you're responding in this way—opening yourself up to spending the time and energy necessary for action—then it's almost certain that you genuinely care. You're not just being nice. You actually want to know what's going on in another person's life.

Second, the question gives us hope...*in ourselves*. It suggests that, despite all the suffering and pain in our world, we as human beings haven't yet given up on each other. In situations that are characterized by hopelessness and suffering, every little indicator of hope and healing— every ray of sunshine—is important to recognize and nurture. Small steps are usually how big change happens, and not some one-time, epic event like a lightning bolt from heaven. It reminds me of Gandalf in *The Fellowship of the Ring:*

> Some believe it is only great power that can hold evil in check.
> But that is not what I have found. I have found that it is
> the small everyday deeds of ordinary folks that keep the darkness
> at bay. Small acts of kindness and love.

Simple questions like "how can I help?" can play a much larger role in a person's life than we imagine. For those who are standing on the brink of despair, it might even save their life. It reminds them that they aren't alone in the world, and pulls them back from the edge.

Third, this question is full of positive potential not just for the person asking, but for the people that they wish to help. The question immediately puts one in the service of another. It attends to a specific person's needs and opens up limitless possibilities for change. It starts a new conversation with new priorities. In short, it plants the seeds for a new path in life.

"What can I do to help?"

It truly is a question we should all be asking every day. Everywhere we look, there are countless people with so much need—and they are longing for us to ask this question and others just like it. And even if the situation isn't dire, everyone wants to improve their lives in some way—and you and I are the ones who have the power to make it happen.

But, *will you?*

Will you put everything else on pause and simply ask, *"What can I do to help?"* (I have a feeling that you wouldn't be reading this book if you hadn't spoken those words at one point!)

My answer to the question always starts with one word.

Love.

1 • LOVE

LOVING LIKE IT MATTERS

I know it seems cliché—and it is certainly overused:

"I *love* pizza."
"I *love* my new job."
"I *love* that movie."

This kind of "love" isn't what I'm talking about—though the incredible popularity of this word *does* tell us something about how central it is for our lives.

The kind of love I'm referring to has a much deeper intensity. It lingers beyond the satisfaction of filling our stomachs or our brains for a few fleeting moments. It goes beyond the surface into a place where it moves us even if we try to stop it. It's a love that can make one person weep uncontrollably and another burst into joyous song.

And yet, it's not an infatuation. It's not lust—a desire to possess, dominate, or consume. Nor is it simply strong desire.[7] No. It is rather a love that can cause a person to leave behind their old life, rise to the occasion, and fight for justice at all costs.

The love that I dream that we would all have towards each other has frequently been called *agápe*.[8] *Agápe* is deeply personal, genuine, and unconditional. In the Christian tradition, it's been said that this is the type of love that God has for human beings. It seeks the good in another for their own sake. The medieval philosopher Thomas Aquinas put it in similar terms, saying that this type of love is to *will the good of another*.[9] When we love someone—when we embody *agápe* —what's good for you becomes what's good for me. Your joy is my joy. Your pain is my pain. Our hearts are drawn together and, in some sense, we become one.

If it sounds radically intense, inclusive, and intimate, *that's because it is*. Consider these famous words:

agápe is patient,
agápe is kind,
it isn't jealous,

it doesn't brag,
it isn't arrogant,
it isn't rude,
it doesn't seek its own advantage,
it isn't irritable,
it doesn't keep a record of complaints,
it isn't happy with injustice,
but it is happy with the truth.
agápe puts up with all things, trusts in all things, hopes for all things,
endures all things.
agápe never fails.[10]

You would think everyone would get excited about something like this!

You would think.

WHERE'S THE LOVE FOR LOVE?

When I discuss and share this type of love with others in answering how they can help, it often makes my audience uncomfortable. People tend to gravitate towards the other types of love that come more naturally to them, like *éros* (associated with romance and sexual passion) or *storgē* (empathy bond, like the love a mother has for her children).[11] When *agápe* is discussed, however, there is a noticeable sense of uneasiness. In fact, when I speak on the Five Ls in various settings, this is the L where I get the most pushback. (Who would have thought "love" would be such a problem!?) The temperature in the room changes and people uncomfortably move around in their seats, all because I've made "love" the focus of attention.

Why does this happen? Don't we live in a society that speaks about "love" every day, pumping out endless movies and songs about it? And aren't many of these "love stories" precisely about finding something *less* shallow, and more *genuine* and *profound*? Furthermore, don't we believe that love is really what people need? How did talking about one of the most universal human experiences become taboo? (Or is it precisely because this kind of love is so *rare* that it stirs people's emotions?)

There's undoubtedly a wide variety of reasons for this discomfort—whether fear that springs from the wounds of death and divorce, or skepticism and hatred towards others that won't allow our clenched fists to open. After all, if love is so valuable to us that people will sometimes kill for it (literally), perhaps it's no wonder when a hush comes over a room simply at its mention.

Love is a sacred thing.

We'll discuss some of these concerns later in the chapter, but whatever the case, I don't mean to judge anyone's reactions. It just strikes me that, at least in today's world, we seem fine with the shallow and trivial kinds of "love," but disagreeable and uneasy about the more serious kind of love that we all crave.

So, I've actually had to soften my approach a little bit and speak of the more general *filía* type love—the strong bond between friends. I reassure my audience that the kind of love we need to have is a brotherly love or a love for humanity. They can then ease into a place of bigger possibilities. For some, this means they don't have to take personal responsibility for something that doesn't have conditions. For others, this means they can hide behind the generic love for humanity as a philosophical idea instead of a personally sacrificial one. (I wish I could just "go big!", but I often don't because I want skeptics to listen, if only for a moment.)

> *...it just strikes me that, at least in today's world, we seem fine with the shallow and trivial kinds of "love," but disagreeable and uneasy about the more serious kind of love that we all crave.*

Nevertheless, this book isn't the *Five Ls (Lite)*. Instead, this book is written with a bold and shameless challenge: to love with reckless abandon—*to love like there is no tomorrow the people who are placed in your path.*

Why "like there is no tomorrow?"

Because there might not *be* tomorrow!

Many of you hardly need reminding about the utter frailty and unpredictability of human life. All of us stand on the edge of death, whether we like it or not. So, what if today was someone's last day, and you were one of the last people to be with them? Wouldn't you want your partner, your son or your daughter, or friend, to feel loved? Isn't that what matters in the end?

Whoa! you're thinking. *This is a lot of weight to put on readers, especially in the first chapter!* Yes, it is. But as I continue to witness a suicide rate of veterans at nearly 20 a day—which excludes countless other suicides— this is not the time for a trite pep talk. It's a sinister reality. So then, why wouldn't it be worth the challenge? Our lives and well-being are at stake— not to mention the lives and well-being of our children, our friends and family, and our communities.

And our life is all that we have.

THE TRIANGLE OF DEATH

This is personal for me. In 2006, 155 men and women, me included, were one Nebraska Army National Guard unit separated from our friends and families for 15 months to serve as part of Operation Iraqi Freedom. Our home, or FOB (Forward Operating Base), for most of the time was located in what was known as the "Triangle of Death." In the heart of the triangle were the cities of Ramadi, Fallujah, and Baghdad.

Our mission in the triangle was to protect ammo and supply convoys driven by contracted U.S. civilians and TCN (Third Country Nationals) who were employed to haul materials in support of the war effort. Our unit, or company, ran an estimated 1,600 combat missions that year, sustaining multiple injuries from IED's (Improvised Explosive Devices). Sadly, my platoon of 30 soldiers also lost one soldier to a roadside bomb on the outskirts of Baghdad.

The injuries and causalities of war were somehow dreadfully anticipated during our deployment. From what I recall, the Department of Defense considered a 15% loss "acceptable." It is the injuries and causalities after war that, to me, have been less acceptable.

Since returning home in 2007, our unit has lost another three to suicide at the time of this writing, one of which was in my squad—one of "my guys." I remember the day I got the news. I was on campus working, and a fellow friend and soldier messaged me that one of our own had died. Just like that. Gone. And like countless other friends and family members who have lost loved ones like this, I'm left wondering, *what on earth could have been done to prevent it?*

It took some time for me to wrestle with the thought of how this brave young man went from standing in the face of a dangerous adversary on the battlefield in the Anbar to lying lifeless on the floor of his home. Was I not there for him? I would have laid my life down for his, but how did I fail him here? Was he trying to reach out? I checked his social media, but it was limited, and of course only showed "good times." Did he message me and I missed it? No messages. Were there any clues that I missed when were last together? Had I listened to him? The list of questions went on and on until I came to the realization that maybe I could not have stopped this senseless death. Then another thought came to me: maybe starting right now, I could do something about this for the rest of my fellow soldiers and other people whom I love.

Perhaps you have felt this way before, too. There are people all around us today living in their "triangle of death," disoriented by what appears to be nothing more than needless suffering, unstoppable public evil, and a world of arbitrary distinctions. So I believe the challenge to *simply and intentionally love* is hardly unjustified.

These people in our lives are waiting and looking for someone to love them. That someone isn't someone *else*.

That someone is *you, and me.*

THE LOGIC OF LOVE

Before looking at what it means to love, we really should ask a more fundamental question.

Why?

For anyone who has "fallen in love," it's a silly question to ask "why?" It just happens. We love because we want to, or sometimes even when we *don't* want to! However, as you might know from experience, authentic love eventually requires more than attraction or inertia. Especially when our partner or friend has been traumatized or hurt and life just isn't the same; loving gets challenging. We find ourselves losing sight of the bigger picture, and begin asking "why?"

This may be especially true today for the millennial and Z generations. The big struggle seems to be *meaninglessness.*[12] Never mind *who* or *how* we love, *why love at all?* It's important then, to at least clear the table and remind ourselves about how and why loving isn't just a chasing after the wind. I certainly don't have a monopoly on this subject, but I do want to offer some provisional answers to this question.

First (and perhaps most obvious), *we love because we all need it, and it's what we would want for ourselves.* Hence, the Silver Rule, "Don't do unto others what you would not have them do unto you," and the Golden Rule, "Do unto others as you would have them do unto you." This kind of proverbial wisdom has been around for thousands of years for good reasons. It assumes that people *need and want* love, which is certainly true. (Has there ever been *too much* love in the world?) And it contends that our love for others is determined by what kind of love we want and need for ourselves. In other words, loving is the *right* thing to do. It is our *responsibility* as human beings towards each other.

But there is another reason why it's important to love, which is the more pragmatic reason that extends out from our responsibility: we love because healthier and happier people around us means *we* can be healthier and happier.

we love because healthier and happier people around us means we can be healthier and happier.

No one truly lives in isolation. We live in communities and depend on each other, even when we try not to. That's how we're made, and how human civilization survives. So, if more and more flourish, then their flourishing will eventually come to make our lives flourish as well. Conversely, if we're surrounded by suffering people, it becomes more and more likely that we will suffer.

Have you ever heard of the saying, "what goes around comes

around?" It's kind of like that. Sociologists (and economists)[13] have noted that "poverty is a problem for everyone, not just for the poor." A fair example of this is what happened in industrial England. At first, hardly anyone with power cared about the intense suffering of factory workers.[14] But then, disease broke out, and attitudes changed:

> Many middle-class citizens were quite willing to support the public health reforms of men like Chadwick because of their fear of cholera. Outbreaks of this deadly disease had ravaged Europe in the early 1930s and late 1840s and were especially rampant in the overcrowded cities. A single wave of cholera in 1832 killed 32,000 people in Paris and another 7,000 in London. As city authorities and wealthier residents became convinced that filthy conditions and poor sewage helped spread the disease, they began to support the call for new public health measures.[15]

Many people were thinking, "well as long as I'm taken care of, I don't have to worry about everybody else." Have you ever thought that way, or known someone who does? As popular as it is, that's just not how the world works.[16] In interconnected communities, it's not so easy to just say "that's their problem" — especially after the coronavirus pandemic of 2020 (social distancing can save lives!). In the end, there isn't some generic "they" that we can continually separate ourselves from.[17] "We're all in this together."

This means we have to *learn compassion*. Compassion is love in response to someone else's suffering or situation. Compassion comes more naturally for empathetic people. They can enter into a person's experience and feel their pain. For others, empathy is more difficult. Detachment and aloofness are easier. Trauma sometimes aggravates empathy because we build up walls of protection. "You may minimize your pain and pretend that you are fine when you aren't. Or you may wear armor around your most vulnerable feelings. You may also protect yourself by pushing away those who care about you when they get too close."[18] Suffice it to say, other people's hurt is an *indicator* for us to step up and respond. Screaming for help makes someone's pain obvious and difficult to ignore. But what about a person's silence, irritability, or changing the subject? Can we see that there might be pain and suffering underneath this—or do we just ignore it and assume that person just didn't get enough sleep last night?

Whatever the case, it remains a fact that without loving others, we're only hurting ourselves. When others are loved, it is more likely that I'll be loved in return. "If one part suffers, all the parts suffer with it; if one part gets the glory, all the parts celebrate with it."[19] Everyone benefits from a more flourishing community.

...without loving others, we're only hurting ourselves...Everyone benefits from a more flourishing community.

Does this mean we should love simply to benefit ourselves in the long run? No. Again, you don't even know if you'll be alive in the "long run!" Even if you did know, we have ethical principles to guide us in questionable situations, and that loving is the right thing to do.

Note that all of this isn't a theory of how love *should* work. It's a statement of fact about how love *does* work. Consider these real-life case studies:

An Amish community forgives a man who shot and killed their schoolgirls. A South African president invites his jailor of twenty-seven years to stand at his side during his inauguration. A Palestinian woman who has lost her son in a terrorist bombing takes in an Israeli boy and raises him as a Jew. A violated gardener befriends an angry boy and teaches him how to grow roses. These exemplars simmer with the miraculous.[20]

This is to mention nothing of major biographies of those who loved powerfully and effectively—from Mother Theresa, to Ghandi, or to Jesus of Nazareth. These people changed the world. *Love is real.*

In the end, then, there are countless *reasons* why we should love each other.[21] The only challenge now is, *how?*

This is a more significant question than it first appears.

While spiritual teachers and advocates of the common good increasingly call for compassion [and love], seldom does anyone explain precisely how to cultivate it. In the absence of practical guidance, acting compassionately seems a near impossible ideal. Our angers, fears, drives, and aversions burn with primal power. Without a means to tend them, we either succumb to shame at our inevitable failures, or we suppress our repulsions, pretend we don't have them, and force a civility that rings hollow to both others and ourselves.[22]

I couldn't agree more, and that's why the rest of this chapter focuses on the "how" question at the most fundamental level.

LEARNING TO LOVE

Hopefully by this point you're thinking, *OK, so I have chosen that "yes," I will love the people that come into my path. But how?* Do you find it odd as you say that? "How do I love?" I know I did as I wrote it. "*How* do I love?" and moreover, "How do I love *well*?"

It really begins with *active and conscious selflessness*. We must start with a basic awareness that we are not the center of the universe, and that we exist largely to serve others—especially those in great need.

In my observations, longevity in marriage is marked by selflessness. People who speak of great love often speak of the humility and selflessness of a great love received. To be selfless, in short, is to turn away from a constant inward focus to instead habitually honor someone above yourself. This is something I have come to learn as I served 21 years in the military and nearly 10 years as a police officer, on top of my time as a pastor: *great love comes with great sacrifice.*

I should note here that the language of "sacrificial love" has fallen into disrepute—and not without reason. For some, it brings up images of a bloody ritual in the ancient world. For others, it is the language used to justify an abusive and manipulative relationship. "Sacrifice" for an abused spouse might mean enduring another year of physical violence. That's obviously not what I'm talking about, and certainly not what I'm encouraging!

When I say "great love comes with great sacrifice," I simply mean that the love isn't arbitrary, without risk, and without a cost. We are *invested* in a person in a way that calls upon our own personal resources—and instead of dreading these costs, we are *willing* to give them up. This kind of selflessness, then, is vital and energetic, not draining and oppressive. It is central for deep and sustainable relationships.

As you can imagine, this kind of positive power and energy has obstacles. Perhaps the biggest obstacle in the way of such selflessness is *pride.* To truly love, pride must be subdued.

Here, we find another curious use of language. Think for a moment about how "pride" is frequently used in the following phrases:

> *When I say "great love comes with great sacrifice," I simply mean that the love isn't arbitrary, without risk, and without a cost. We are* invested *in a person that calls upon our own personal resources...*

"*Take pride in your work.*"
"*Take pride in your appearance.*"
"*Take pride in your country.*"

The keyword here isn't pride.

It's *take.*

Pride always seems to take, but if you think about humility, that is about *giving away.* Putting away our pride opens the door to selflessness and selflessness to loving well. To reiterate the quote from earlier in this chapter: "*agápe* ...isn't jealous, it doesn't brag, it isn't arrogant, it isn't rude, it doesn't seek its own advantage, it isn't irritable, it doesn't keep a record of complaints..." In other words, love is all about focusing on "the other"—the person outside of myself that I can serve.

PRESS PAUSE

The second key to loving well—and I think it is only second to selflessness because you can't have this without being selfless—is *patience.*

Our world is impatient! Let me say it again for emphasis: *our world is impatient.* This is especially true for those who happen to live in the exciting world of the twenty-first century (which happens to be all of us!).

In many ways, this strange and busy world *rewards* impatience. "Go-getters" get all the pay raises, not the skeptical or cautious. And in some ways, the world punishes those who stop, think, wait, care, and recover as long as is needed. (After all, such "unproductive" time is considered "wasted" time.)

Take grieving the loss of a loved one, for example. Anyone who has witnessed death and burial ceremonies of some cultures outside the western world knows how rushed our way of grieving can be. In places like the U.S., the body is quickly covered up and stowed away almost instantly, a funeral is usually within about a 7-10 days (with the burial just hours after that), and maybe we take off a week from work. Then that's it. Back to our routine. Contrast that with some Native American traditions, where the body was clothed and treated as alive in the place of its death for up to a year, followed by burial and then a multi-day service. Or consider Islam, where it is common for widows to mourn for four months and ten days. Eastern Orthodox commemorate the "40th day after death." Jewish traditions have thirty-day (*shloshim*) and twelve-month (*shneim asar chodesh*) mourning procedures. And so on. The more and more modernized and westernized the world becomes, it seems the more and more "efficient" we get at dying and detaching.

As a result, the more and more incompetent we are to be patient and attend to the needs of our hearts and souls. (Note that I say all this as a terribly impatient person. I'm typing as fast as I can so I can get this book out to people who I've already sold it to!)

In many ways, our lack of patience is really a product of our ability to get what we want *right now*. It doesn't matter what it is — information, products, entertainment, advice, food. It can be delivered to you in minutes. Just stop and listen to ourselves:

"I don't have time to read books…"
"It's been over two days already; where's my stuff from Amazon!?"

"Because of the line at the grocery store, I had to wait *ten minutes* just to get out and..."

"This red light is taking *forever...*"

We're all absurd! And it's no wonder, then, that some of the best-selling books on personal, spiritual and mental health are about *slowing down and living in the now.* It reminds me of something the great philosopher and mathematician Blaise Pascal once wrote centuries ago:

> Let each one examine [their] thoughts, and [they] will find them all occupied with the past and the future. We scarcely ever think of the present; and if we think of it, it is only to take light from it to arrange the future. The present is never our end. The past and the present are our means; the future alone is our end. So we never live, but we hope to live; and, as we are always preparing to be happy, it is inevitable we should never be so.[23]

Patience can help us live contently in the now instead of forcing the future into the present. It is also central for the healing of the traumatized:

> For real change to take place, the body needs to learn that the danger has passed and to live in the reality of the present.[24]

Even though we have been sold this idea of "love at first sight" and instant gratification, love really is a game of patience. It's a rough analogy, but I often think about how infatuation is the kind of love that is microwaved. You can have it really quick, but the end product usually isn't anything impressive. When I think of patience and love, I think of a slow-cooker. When you put something in a slow-cooker and let it simmer for hours, there is a certain richness to the food. (The smells and flavors of the dish can be almost emotionally described!) In the end, food cooked with care and patience—"with love!"—provides something genuine that lasts in both enjoyment and nourishment.

Love that comes from patience can produce nourishment for the soul.

Similarly, love that comes from patience can produce nourishment for the soul. Who doesn't want or need that?

WHAT LOVE LOOKED LIKE FOR ME

My deployment to Iraq was a great test of my wife (Jodi's) patience. I told her when I left that I wouldn't call often. In fact, I told her I would only call and talk to her and the kids just once a month while I was away for the 15 months. We talked about this, and I let her know that hearing her voice and the voices of our kids would just be…too much for me. I just had to stay focused as a squad leader. I needed to make sure the mission was accomplished, that my troops and I made it home. Jodi was working full time along with parenting our teenaged son and preteen daughter, and I knew that by doing this, I was asking her for even more.

She didn't skip a beat. She understood the situation. She was patient when I wasn't able to call on the day we had planned to talk, and patient if I didn't respond to an email because one of my combat missions went days longer than I had anticipated (War can be so rude sometimes!) And after that, she still had patience to then listen as I recounted my time at war. Never once did she make me feel guilty for going away for so long and leaving her at home with all the responsibilities of taking care of our little family. Through her patience, I could vividly see her great love for me.

I speak from the context of my memories about the toughness and individualism exhibited by my partner in life. I am also highly aware though that everything between Jodi and I wasn't perfect. We are people, after all, and not one of us can claim perfection. Being gone so long, there were undoubtedly things around the house that needed our attention, as did our marriage. Yet she went out of her way to give me the space I needed to lead my squad, even if everything wasn't just fine at home. She had more to deal with than broken doors and peeling paint after my homecoming.

She had to deal with *me*.

Immediately upon my return, she could instinctively tell that I had experienced events that had changed me. I was no longer the pre-war man that she had married and I didn't like this any more than she did.

I came home with some very telltale signs of Post-Traumatic Stress Disorder. But, *amazingly,* even when I couldn't sleep in our bed because it was just too big and I didn't feel safe, or when I couldn't stand the Independence Day celebrations because the loud cracks and booms were too much to bear—no matter what I was like after returning from the battlefield, she chose to love me unconditionally. With grace and strength, she stood patiently by me and carved out an environment that allowed me to begin to heal.

Throughout this difficult journey I've learned this: loving well is, at the very least, a combination of selflessness and patience; it is an opportunity and a responsibility for you and me to help those in our path who have struggled with the stress of trauma.

...if you want to have long-lasting, positive effects on traumatized loved-ones, selflessness and patience is absolutely essential.

These aren't exactly values, virtues, or practices that our world holds highly right now—no matter what kind of relationship you're in. But if you want to have long-lasting, positive effects on traumatized loved ones, selflessness and patience are absolutely essential.

STILL WORRIED ABOUT LOVE?

For those of you who find the first L troubling, there is, in fact, good reason for this, and I want to briefly focus on that now. At some point, you will need to decide for yourself if the risks of radical love overshadow your renewed knowledge about it.

The first and most obvious reason to be worried is that *loving is hard.*

How do we refrain from doing what is hateful to another when someone treats us with hateful distain?
How do we care with unwavering impartiality when tension, exhaustion, and unending demands are sustained burdens on our spirits?

How do we love our enemies—[someone who has] abused us, for example—when their impassive non-repentance renders mercy obscene and downright irresponsible?

How do we love our enemies when, driven by perfectionism and our own castigation, our enemies are ourselves?

How do we love our enemies when the people who most repel and infuriate us are our very own children, partners, and parents?[25]

Some situations may not be difficult at all, while others may seem impossible. Whatever your situation is, there's no getting around it: the project of love is not for the faint-hearted.

A second challenge is related: *loving can be dangerous*. It always involves risk. Loving someone means opening up your heart to the real possibility of hurt. Loving *well* opens it further until we are completely vulnerable. Who enjoys being completely vulnerable? It's worse than streaking down Main Street!

I recently read a book titled *Backlash* by George Yancy.[26] The book responds to the backlash he received from writing the *New York Times* essay "Dear White America," where he asked white people to avail themselves to change by being vulnerable in the debates and social problems surrounding systemic racism. He contends that change can't really happen until we open ourselves up to possible hurt.

He's right—and this isn't easy. It takes serious courage and strength to expose ourselves in this way. Most of us have been hurt at a *heart level* when it comes to love. In fact, so many traumas experienced by people come from trusting the ones who we love. My trust has been broken from past relationships just like all of you, and the question we have is all the same: *How can I then open myself back up to love? Is it worth the risk?*

Answering this is tough, especially since loving and losing trust is often a source of trauma. Even the idea of "forgive and forget" becomes an obstacle. Consider the following story:

Maria's stepfather sexually abused her throughout her childhood. After years of therapy, she has created a stable life. More than a survivor, she is thriving—she is married, studying women's health, and raising a daughter of her own. For nearly ten years, however, she has refused to be in the same city with the man who violated her. Her religious friends have been little help, admonishing her to forgive and let go, telling her that her resentment will eat her from the inside out. Yet even the thought of him enrages her; the very word *forgiveness* makes her want to scream. Now, her younger brother is getting married and wants her daughter to be the flower girl. Both he and their mother implore Maria to bring her family to the wedding. She is genuinely torn. She loves her brother, and her daughter would be thrilled. But that man sitting next to her mother ignites a fury inside her that wants to torch the entire event. How does she care for both herself and her family when her abuser remains present and unrepentant?

How indeed.[27]

The late Rachel Held Evans provided some important qualifiers on this complex topic, and they serve as helpful guardrails:

1. Forgiveness does not require staying in an abusive situation;
2. Forgiveness does not require accepting empty apologies or trusting the bully/abuser;
3. Grace does not require remaining silent about bullying and abuse;
4. Forgiveness and grace do not preclude justice or demand superficial reconciliation.[28]

With such conditions in mind (to whatever extent they are relevant), it remains vital to *lean* in the direction of hope, and where appropriate, make room for the possibility of authentic forgiveness, which can bring new life to relationships. If we can do this—a big "if" to be sure—we may create new space in our hearts for love and vulnerability.

> Forgiveness—letting go of negative emotions toward whoever or whatever has done us harm, and toward ourselves for the real or imagined damage we have done to ourselves or to others—is a powerful ally in trauma recovery. But we need to know when and how to make this alliance...forgiveness and justice are not necessarily opposed. Forgiveness is far easier if we feel justice has been done...

> Ultimately, though, we embrace forgiveness because it is such a powerful

force for healing us and making us whole....It purges us of resentment's emotional and spiritual poison and its high levels of biological stress...A number of scientific studies have shown that in forgiving others we become more relaxed. Chronic pain subsides, and high blood pressure goes down. Our mood improves. We feel more optimistic. Combat veterans who are more capable of forgiveness have fewer symptoms of post-traumatic stress disorder.[29]

A broader understanding of forgiveness isn't even for the person whom I have forgiven but for us.[30] When we carry hate or offense, the weight and the mass of each of those stories and dynamics is bore by us, not only by the perpetrator of our trauma. By making room for forgiveness, it's possible to take back what was stolen from me in trauma and I'm allowed to then have the capacity to love someone else when they are in desperate need of it. For, "If we do not *transform* our pain, we will most assuredly *transmit* it—usually to those closest to us."[31]

Loving well means consciously and intentionally partaking in the work of *transformation* instead of transmission, and that specifically requires patience and selflessness.

A BRIEF WORD TO DUDES

I'm a dude, and most combat veterans are dudes, and there's some unique challenges that I think we that affect us and everyone else, so I want to address that now.

For many men, loving well looks weak or effeminate. Especially in western culture, men are supposed to be consistently masculine (whatever that might mean) and fairly absent emotionally. Some argue that there are good reasons for this, and important social benefits. These arguments range anywhere from being able to effectively fight in war, to having the ability to kill grizzly bears that wander into a camp, or (most importantly!) shooting dozens of cute little bunnies for a starving family in the woods.

OK, set aside the bludgeoning of cute little bunnies for a moment and just notice how these other engagements require love. If I go to war, there must be love of something or someone. If I wrestle a grizzly, I obviously have a more important reason than my own life in doing so. "No one has greater love than to give up one's life for one's friends."[32] So even the positive aspects of "masculine traits" (heroism, strength, courage) could be expressions of love.

More importantly, these stereotypes and attitudes in their full colors tend to forge a hardened heart that makes it particularly difficult for men to (a) articulate their own internal emotions to others and (b) open themselves up to the possibility of intimate relationships. How so?

First, it makes empathy itself seem cowardly. Infantry soldiers might be the most deeply affected this way because they're mentally forced to dehumanize and detach from those who are being killed. (They have to, otherwise pulling the trigger would be impossible.)[33] And I don't know if it's American militarism, empire mentalities, or just a century of bad movies, but empathy is actually considered a *problem* for almost everyone these days. One psychologist has actually written a book entitled *Against Empathy*,[34] while another (wildly popular) speaks of "too much empathy" and "compassion as a vice."[35] Combined with the rise of various leaders and politicians known for being authoritarian (and frequently abusive) tough-guys, being mean and heartless is now considered cool. (This problem was recently featured by a historian in a book titled *Jesus and John Wayne*.[36]) To put it bluntly, *the kind of radical love I'm advocating is almost considered a threat to society*.[37] Our world is telling us that love, empathy, and compassion is for the *weak* as much as it is telling us that patience *isn't* a virtue.[38]

> One study of American students published in *Personality and Social Psychology Review* revealed that levels of empathy in this demographic fell by 48 percent between 1979 and 2009. Possible causes of the growing empathy gap include increasing materialism, changing parenting methods and the digital echo chamber, in which people anchor themselves in close-knit groups of like-minded people... The *Global Risks Report* highlights that while online connections can be empathetic, research suggests that the degree of empathy is six times weaker than for real-world interactions.[39]

Is it any wonder why so many people seem irritated, angry, depressed, and suicidal? Not for this camper. I really believe this is a backwards-looking orientation that intensifies our problems. Especially in the twenty-first century, just moments after the bloodiest and most violent century in the history of the world,[40] I really don't think society's problem is "too much compassion." It is unfortunate that we actually have to fight for the meaningfulness of empathic love!

Second, these hyper-masculine attitudes reduce "strength" to assertiveness or brute force, when in fact, strength can be found in restraint, complex thinking that requires patience, or being able to withhold judgment when it's extremely difficult not to. Sometimes listening up and being influenced requires as much fortitude and courage as speaking up and influencing. For some college students, sitting in front of a professor and letting them shape your ideas about the world is like letting a tarantula slowly crawl up your ear and into your brain. That's some serious discipline there! I know some people whose choice to speak to their parents after many years took more courage and strength out of them than any other act in their life. For others, a phone call, a move to another country, or voluntarily letting go of a relationship can be an act of immeasurable fortitude. The fact is, (a) strength comes in many forms, and there is no reason to prioritize one kind of strength over all others, (b), it's absurd to suggest that all men simply and inherently have a monopoly on strength, and (c) simply put, "vulnerability is strength,"[41] not weakness. More on this later.

...strength can be found in restraint, complex thinking that requires patience, or being able to withhold judgment when it's extremely difficult not to. Sometimes listening up and being influenced requires as much fortitude and courage as speaking up and influencing.

Third, these attitudes (often called "toxic masculinity" —yes, it's real) train men to view everyone and everything else as passive objects to be rescued, conquered, or consumed instead of viewing and treating them as living beings. This can cause all kinds of relational problems. In its worst form, it facilitates violence. A recent study covering over seventy-five countries found (among other things) that "almost a third of men and women think it's acceptable for a man to beat his wife."[42] Whoa! This was from 2020—covering a geography equivalent to 80% of the world population! Meanwhile, months later, 007 (Sean Connery) passes away with mass admiration from millions—an actor who made a notorious case for beating women during a public interview with Barbara Walters.[43]

It's funny, right?

No, it's not. We've got a long ways to go.

Don't get me wrong: there's nothing problematic about being disciplined, principled, bold, or even protective and assertive. All of that is necessary for defensive operations in the Middle East (…and for training dogs…and fighting the traffic to get to work). But there are probably good reasons behind the fact that veteran (*and* non-veteran) suicides are disproportionately male,[44] or that about a third of male police officers (often trained to be aggressive) beat their wives.[45] Perhaps most obviously, it is considered dishonorable or weak for male soldiers or police officers to go in for counseling. They're often encouraged by comrades to "ball up" or to "just drink it off" (as if that would help; more on this later).

This is where the logic of love is upside down, because *the courageous and bold thing to do is to "man-up," swallow your pride, and seek help instead of running from it.* Real men know how to love and how to be loved. They can face their suffering and open up in front of another human being, taking the risk of not knowing what will happen. Or, they can quickly and conveniently stuff it away month after month.

> Many of us…have learned or decided that emotions are dangerous, and likely self-indulgent as well. Our parents have suppressed or denied their own feelings in the name of toughness or proper behavior, or looking good or being strong for others. They—and later, teachers and bosses—may have dismissed our feelings as distractions from academic achievement, impediments to superior work performance, flaws rather than valued facets of our character….[But] our emotions are not our

enemies. They can, in fact, be friends and allies on our healing journey.[46]

Ever since Roman civilization, men have been taught that being "soft" — seeking help, loving with compassion, and being slow to use force (if ever) — is dishonorable. But it's not. It's just part of being alive and being a decent human. Indeed, being stiff and closed-off from influence only aggravates the pain and suffering underlying trauma.

So, I close this section with some words from the *Tao Te Ching* (yes, perhaps an odd place given its gender stereotypes); I hope readers affected by a rigid heart and stiff emotions will dwell on these words:

Men are born soft and supple;
dead, they are stiff and hard.
Plants are born tender and pliant;
dead, they are brittle and dry.

Thus whoever is stiff and inflexible
is a disciple of death.
Whoever is soft and yielding
is a disciple of life.

The hard and stiff will be broken.
The soft and supple will prevail.[47]

HANG-UPS

As we wrap up this chapter, there are two other hang-ups on loving well that I should mention. The first is *misunderstanding*.

In my experience, when you're found suddenly loving where you were not before, people sometimes question your authenticity. "What's he or she trying to get by acting this way?" They wonder what your angle is, question your motives, or look for reasons to find something wrong with you. They might even feel intimidated that someone is actually refusing to just accept that there's no hope.

Don't let this throw you off. These are misunderstandings that are best shrugged off with the passing of time and faithful action. If you're "for real," it will become evident to your community and loved ones over time. Look at the big picture: people in your path are praying for someone like you to step into their lives, and that is infinitely more important than rumors, judgmentalism, or maybe your reputation as being "tough." Loving well is worth the risk of being misunderstood.

A second problem is the classic problem of economics: *scarcity*. We have limitations. You're just one person, and there are *so* many people that need love. I've often wondered: what difference is one person's compassion towards others? It's at that point that I'm again reminded of the obvious answer: *it might save a life.*

It all depends on the situation. I came across the following quote the other day, and it really sums up how I think we might approach this problem:

> All people should be loved equally. But you cannot do good to all people equally, so you should take particular thought for those who, as if by lot, happen to be particularly close to you in terms of place, time, and any other circumstances.
>
> Suppose that you had plenty of something which had to be given to someone in need of it but could not be given to two people, and you met two people, neither of whom had a greater need or a closer relationship to you than the other: you could do nothing more just than to choose by lot the person to whom you should give what could not be given to both.[48]

So often when it comes to a need, we get overwhelmed by the universality of it all. Hunger and famine in third world countries, water needs in Africa, genocide, military occupations and needless war, record-breaking wildfires, and the list literally goes on and on. Our era is the first in history where we can be globally aware of what's happening in real time. You just pull out your phone. But this brave new world of instantaneous information poses a new challenge, because it's obviously good to be aware of how great the need is. On the other hand, if it causes you to freeze or sink into hopelessness, then it isn't good. (I talk more about this in the section on hope in "Concluding Reflections.")

My suggestion is simple: *take care of your immediate sphere of influence*— your work, your school, your family, your church, your neighbors, etc. You already have a head start this way and don't have to get overwhelmed with all the people and things "out there."

You have a beautiful and precious gift to give those closest to you. *You're in their lives for a reason.* It's time to live like it.

CONCLUSION

I can't stress enough the importance of love in the process of healing for people in trauma or people who are contemplating suicide. It's like talking about the importance of water in a pool for an Olympic swimmer moving from one end to the other. It's the whole thing. Life is impossible without it. And of all of the things I will discuss in this book, this L, *L. O. V. E.*, is key. Without it, nothing else will work effectively. You can master all of the other Ls in the chapters ahead, but they will have no foundation and blow away with the newest fad of trauma-help how-to's.

You and I have the chance to take a leap into a place that really makes a difference. If you embrace this fully and are aware of your own lack of it, you know what I am speaking about. If there was one substance you wish were bottled and you could take to ease your own suffering, you know that *Love* would be on the side of that bottle and the directions would read, "take one whenever you need it, because it is good for what ails you." Love is an anchor when things are rocky, and it can be the thing that sets us free when we are feeling trapped. It's the most universal and powerful human experience for good reasons. Anyone can do this; we can't let it go to waste!

In the end, love is a choice—and it's a serious one. It isn't something that just comes with breathing, at least not as I have described it. It is a choice that comes with ramifications. When you make the choice to love and to do it well, you must go in with your eyes wide open.

And when we do take this bold step, there is no limit to what can change.

QUESTIONS FOR REFLECTION

1. Do you find yourself guarded when it comes to loving someone? What causes this in your life?

2. What connections do you see between forgiveness and love? Why is this important for you to understand based on what you know about love?

3. What was an episode of your life where you felt profoundly loved? What do you think made it so profound and moving?

4. What was an episode of your life that tested your patience in loving someone? Were you aware of how this got in the way of loving them, and did this influence your actions? Why or why not?

5. Recall the "Golden Rule." How is following the Golden Rule impossible without empathy?

6. Radical love is *inclusive*. In first century Palestine, it was a big deal for people to love, accept, and dignify women, lepers, children, eunuchs, and Samaritans. What would this kind of radical, inclusive love look like today? What people and groups are shameful to you that you find difficult to love—people you would feel ashamed to have at your dinner table? "Love your enemies" we have heard. Could you do this?

7. Professor Brené Brown has sometimes focused on a question that can get us to think empathetically and compassionately and develop our emotional intelligence. Think about someone you find difficult to love that's in your life—people you wish would get their act together somehow. And now, think long and hard about the question: *Do you think they are doing the best they can?*

2

LISTEN

Listen, I am alone at a crossroads, I'm not at home in my own home
And I've tried and tried, To say what's on my mind, You should have known,
oh Now I'm done believin' you,
You don't know what I'm feelin' I'm more than what You've made of me,
followed the voice you gave to me But now I've gotta find my own.
You should have listened.

"Listen"
BEYONCÉ

STAND AT EASE

It's been said that "you have two ears and only one mouth for a reason." I agree, and the importance of listening is visible all around us.

In the world of higher education that I experience every day, there is a great deal of buzz about *listening*. Some of it has to do with listening to various groups that have never really had a microphone in society—minorities, the oppressed, the colonized, etc. This is directly relevant to educators and leaders in the academy—as the great African-American philosopher and prophet Cornel West declared, "The vocation of the intellectual is to let suffering speak, let victims be visible, and let social misery be put on the agenda of those in power."[49]

But there's also talk about the methods of listening. Some time ago I remember learning about *"active* listening." If you want to learn how to listen, there's an endless library of self-help books published on the subject. In the Army, there is specific training for listening. In fact, when in formation, there is a popular command you're probably familiar with called "Stand at ease."

To the untrained ear, this command might only mean "relax" or "chill out." But to those of us who have served, we know this command is actually the opposite of chill: it means "pay attention!" The preparatory command, which brings you to a place of paying attention, are the words "stand" and "at." (You are already standing so there is no need to get up from a sitting position.) The last part of the command tells you *how* you are to stand: at "ease." This simple form allows only your head to move back and forth in order to follow the speaker in front of the formation. With the remainder of one's body at rest, the soldier is able to pay full attention with their eyes and ears to understand what's being said.

Why such drama for listening? Because in combat operations, each soldier in a unit has a specific duty in understanding the orders as they are given, and what the rest of the unit understands can mean the difference between life and death—yours or your buddy's life, that is. This is the one moment you don't want to be day-dreaming.

LEARNING TO LISTEN

I wonder sometimes if we all could take a lesson in listening from the Army. What if we thought about listening in a different way? What if we took it seriously and thought about listening as a life-or-death choice? After all, things get really chaotic when people who need help aren't heard. "Riots are the voice of the unheard," as Martin Luther King said. Perhaps something similar applies to our hurting friends—the chaos within them gets worse the more that they feel unheard.

The fact is, listening is the bridge to empathy and central to the path of almost any kind of healing. But here is how most of us "listen"—and it's not because we have ill intent (quite the contrary), but it's just what tends to happen...and happens all the time:

We listen with the intent of talking.

"Listening" in this case is just a means to an end, which is ultimately to put the spotlight on ourselves. *This isn't actually listening.*

Listening means subordinating yourself to the speaker and entering into their experience as an end in itself. Whether you "get" to talk afterwards is irrelevant. That's why there is both some truth and untruth about the

> *Listening means subordinating yourself to the speaker and entering into their experience as an end in itself.*

metaphor of *"paying"* attention. Listening *is* costly. It places a demand on us. It takes time and energy. (Ask any pastor or therapist!) But on the other hand, it's not a form of currency. Listening isn't like math where if I listen a certain amount, this entitles me to the same amount of speaking (though it is true good conversations tend to be reciprocal). Good listening has no intention of "payback." And if we turn listening into a *ticket* for our own speaking, our mind isn't actually focused on what words are being spoken to us but on what we think our best response will be.

This kind of response is typically called *advice*. As you may have noticed, there is no lack of advice in today's world. Anyone can start a blog and become a fee-charging "life coach" overnight. The advice of male know-it-alls is so bad we've created a new word for it ("man-splaining"). I'm as guilty for this problem as much as anyone, so I'm not wearing the proverbial halo in this situation. We all want to help, so we think of ways of doing that, and giving advice often seems practical and caring. But if we really want to help—especially those who need a voice—instead of *offering* something, we should be *accepting* whatever we're given.

This is, first, because listening itself is in some ways a gift that we give others. We should be viewing each opportunity as a chance to help someone else. Second, listening allows us to get to know the person speaking to us, which is what we would want for ourselves (refer back to chapter 1 on Love and the Golden Rule). And when someone is talking about their life or situation, it's obviously important to them. *They are giving you a piece of their life.*

Seeing it this way, I can't help but notice the selfishness in my own habits and responses to people. I am actually more worried about how my response is going to be received, or how I will sound when saying it, than I am about what the other person is saying and experiencing. That's a problem.

There's an important caveat to this whole discussion, however: *people usually know when you are listening and when you're not.* Unless they're ultra-motor-mouths that only talk talk talk (and I've met my share of those...), they can sense when your *mhmm*s and *oh yeah*s and *really?*s are just auto-pilot responses, and when they are genuine engagement. (And then, sometimes people don't even try. One of my biggest pet peeves is when someone asks me a question and when I respond, they're looking somewhere else as if I had said nothing. It's like, *hey!, you asked me a question but my response is apparently so far down on your "importance scale" that you can't even acknowledge it in the first place?*)

So much of listening really is in our body language. You can try to hide body language expressions like doing your best to look at the person speaking to you, or leaning in while they speak. But there is a lot of study on *nonverbal* communication, and how we say things in our body language that we're not even aware of. Some of those things can destroy the mutuality and respect required for genuine listening and a heart-to-heart conversation.

Sociologists have come to recognize a subset of this disruptive, nonverbal communication as "microaggressions."[50] Consider when a white woman, for example, unconsciously clutches her purse when walking past a Black man. (The racist idea underneath here is that "Black men are thieves.") Or consider when a man at a business meeting habitually touches the forearm of the woman next to him each time she talks—which is a condescending gesture asserting that she is small and he is in control. (The sexist idea underneath here

Microaggression: a comment or action that subtly and often unconsciously or unintentionally expresses a prejudiced attitude toward a member of a marginalized group (such as a racial minority) (Merriam Webster)

is that "women are weak" or "women should let the men do the talking, because men are better at leadership.") Microaggressions are obviously more than a rude gesture. They create an oppressive world. They regularly remind people of their social position and encourage people to behave in super-ordinate and subordinate ways. But at the very least, they cause a breakdown in communications because they reveal and embody our prejudices and value system. This disjunction undermines mutuality. (It's hard to have a real conversation with someone when you're subordinating or belittling them the whole time!)

How can we change these kinds of habits and inclinations? It's not easy; it's not something that you can change without some really deep soul searching—and practice.[51] But we can at least be aware of these dynamics when entering into those important conversations. Our words and our hidden assumptions matter, and they may ultimately need adjustment.

Besides our hidden prejudices, there are also those times that we listen with preconceived notions, and instead of helping us interpret how things are, they just get in the way. We all have a mental grid that determines what we think is possible or probable. So, often enough, when approaching a person or situation, we have already told ourselves that we know what the person will be asking or wanting and even how they will ask for it. We live out the *scripts and stories* we've learned from society.

One day Jodi was walking to the grocery store and saw a man near one of the intersections on the way there. He appeared to be homeless in his dress and how he held himself, and she could see him trying to talk to people passing by, but no one would stop. She initially thought, like many of us, that the man would want something (money, food, alcohol perhaps), so she thought about going a different direction. But she crossed the street and the man approached her.

"I was wondering if you could help me get home. I have been wondering around for about three hours and I can't remember how to get to my house."

With no reason not to help, Jodi assisted him in finding his bearings and got him pointed in the right direction. No problem.

Later on, she told me how she was anticipating the awkwardness of encountering the more stereotypical beggar. He would want money, and she normally doesn't carry cash. But once she actually listened, it wasn't that at all. It was someone who needed a different kind of help right away, and because of that, she was able to give him everything he needed simply because of two things: (1) she chose to question the popular script about what would happen, and (2) she chose to listen well.

The filtered, biased kind of "listening" would have produced a different result. It causes a person to give up before getting to the real issue at hand, makes you avoid the conversation altogether, or pushes you to prepackage your response. In the end, it shuts doors for communication instead of opens them, and therefore shuts the door to the possibility of change.

Virtually every person contemplating suicide is stuck telling themselves—and then living out—the same scripts. We talk to ourselves in our heads and say how things are, and live accordingly, and do this over and over. Ultimately, those scripts and narratives are some form of hopelessness and being held captive by something too powerful to overcome. Scripts and stories about ourselves are also constructed in words. That's why focusing on language can be so important.

Sometimes we can help by putting words to experiences for our loved ones. You may be talking and then they say, "yes, that's the right word, thank you." Ever have that happen? Other times, however, our use of words can be as entrapping as liberating. Some of my therapist friends are frustrated when other therapists (playing the role of expert) take away the words of clients and replace them with unhelpful scientific terminology and psychobabble, instead of letting clients use their own vocabulary for the problems they have. Our traumatized loved ones should feel safe— and encouraged—to interpret their own experience in their own language.

We cannot live in a world that is not our own, in a world that is interpreted for us by others. An interpreted world is not a home. Part of the terror is to take back our own listening, to use our own voice, to see our own light.[52]

Healing from trauma is a process of *recreating ourselves*. As the author of *The Post-Traumatic Growth Guidebook* puts it: "The transformational work of healing from trauma asks you to embrace change—to live in limbo and stand in the transitional space between the person you have been in the past and the person you are becoming."[53]

So, it's our job as allies, partners, and friends to (a) make sure we're listening enough to identify what those entrapping scripts are, and (b) find and give attention instead to those other stories and voices in a person's life that offer more hope, new possibilities, and a new identity for the road ahead.[54] Asking our loved one about who they want to be and learning about moments in their life where they felt moved in that direction can be pivotal points as you walk the road of darkness together.

But it all starts with genuine listening.

GOOD LISTENING CAN BE INTENSE

As you might imagine, the type of listening that I want to discuss is just like the task of Love: it isn't for the faint of heart, or the "just too busy." It will take time and patience (and we all know that both of these are at a premium in our day-to-day lives).

As a Christian with a background in various ministries, I can't help but connect genuine listening to the classic stories in biblical literature. The more and more I've learned about listening, the more and more I've noticed how Jesus of Nazareth got his hands dirty in the lives of traumatized individuals.[55] While there are lots of legends and myths surrounding the person, it seems that Jesus was not only a remarkable teacher, but a remarkable listener.[56] Virtually nothing is known about him or his teaching until his 30s (he apparently didn't have LinkedIn like me to talk all about his experience!). Then, things got rolling, and he found himself surrounded by a world of violence and hurt. He heard the cry of the poor, the sick, needy, oppressed, and alienated.

And *he attended to it*. His perception and attention ultimately peered into people's souls so deeply that nobody could forget it.[57] In contrast to the religious authorities, who had a filtered grid of "listening" that only served to protect their own interests, Jesus genuinely heard the hearts of people—no matter who it was who came to him. There was no one too ordinary or too broken for him to engage in authentic conversation with, and to begin the process of "binding up the broken-hearted."[58]

You might recall the well-known story of Cain and Abel from the Hebrew scriptures. The story is known for all kinds of reasons, but there's this memorable one-liner that I think just captures it. If you're not familiar with the story, here's my summary: Abel brings a sacrifice to God and God looks on it with favor, but then Cain brings his own sacrifice and God says "this ain't right bro," so Cain gets ticked off so much he eighty-sixes his brother even though it wasn't his fault at all. God then speaks to Cain— and this is the interesting part: "What did you do? The voice of your brother's blood is crying to me from the ground" (Gen 4:10, CEB).

Whoa! This is the kind of listening I'm talking about. *It's where you can hear the pain and suffering and crying of another human being even where there are no tears in sight.*

I should mention that this kind of intuitive listening is particularly helpful when conversations get tense. Sometimes criticism from your loved one has nothing to do with you. Perhaps the person is just under so much stress that they can't contain it anymore, or they don't realize what they're saying through their *feelings* and it comes out in a reckless avalanche. In those tense moments, it's important not to deflect or argue out of it, because that's not what the conversation is really about. It's better to try to reflect in a way that, on the one hand, isn't dismissive, but on the other hand, says "I'm still here with you, and still listening."

You can see then, that this is above and beyond the call of "Stand at ease." It's *intense*. Have you ever tried to listen for a single drop of rain hitting the ground? Have you silenced the noise around you to hear the birds chirping in the morning? Have you worked to eradicate all sounds so you can be attentive to your spouse or partner in the moment that they are sharing something that might change everything?

We might as well say that good listening is *aerobic* listening. It takes energy and our whole body is engaged. As a leading authority on PTSD puts it:

Visiting the past in therapy [or in conversation] should be done while people are, biologically speaking, firmly rooted in the present and feeling as calm, safe, and grounded as possible. ("Grounded" means that you can feel your butt in your chair, see the light coming through the window, feel tension in your calves, and hear the wind stirring the tree outside.) Being anchored in the present while re-visiting the trauma opens the possibility of deeply knowing that the terrible events belong to the past.[59]

PRACTICAL STEPS FOR GENUINE LISTENING

What concrete steps can a person take to mentally and physically prepare them for genuine listening? Because, apart from the first L, this is probably most important to the process of helping someone who has been placed in your path. The L of listening will help to give you the insight you need to be able to do the next three Ls in this book.

First, aerobic listening requires attending to our own bodies, and getting them in order. Consider your feet. We are so, *so* busy these days. We move from place to place constantly—from soccer game to swim meet, to a friend's house, to our parents' house, to work, to school, and so on that our ability to listen almost seems dictated by our feet. Here are a few suggestions.

So *just stand still for a minute.* Get under control and get comfortable. "Plant your feet," if you will, and don't allow your anxious limbs and mobility and schedule to get in the way of your ears. When the only thing on our minds is the next meeting or getting to bed on time, this requires some real mental and *physical self-discipline.* Your speaker—your partner or loved one—needs to know that you aren't going anywhere, and that they are more important than the ordinary events of everyday life. People who have lost hope often need some sign that they're "on your schedule," as it were. That might mean taking some work off, cancelling a meeting, or doing whatever it takes to ensure that a tough conversation finishes as good as it can given the circumstances. Because the fact is, expectations of success and responsibilities that we all bear cause our feet to move almost uncontrollably. We literally have to make a conscience decision to just *stop* and listen.

Second, pay attention to your stomach. If you know that you're going into a real listening session, then good heavens, at least make sure you aren't hungry going in! Hunger, believe it or not, is one of the biggest obstacles to aerobic listening. Grab a snack if you can or whatever is necessary to keep your belly from groaning and tugging at your ears. I know this isn't always possible given the constraints of time, but it's worth trying. You want to be as awake and engaged as possible without having to cut it short.

Third, prepare a space free from distraction. Are you fidgety like me? I always seem to find myself spinning my wedding ring, clicking a pen, or tapping the table. Even though you may not mean it to, sometimes these things can come across as impatience. Prepare for your conversation by putting those kinds of distractions out of reach (unless you really need them to focus, and you're confident that they're not distracting). Put your cell phone on silent and make it disappear. No one wants to tell you their trauma story—or even what they had for dinner last night—while you glance over at the day's (usually unimportant) social media feeds. Don't check the time. In short, cultivate practices and an environment that allows you to keep focus.

The next group of muscles that may be the most important to listening aerobically, apart from your ears, are those two eyes you have in the middle of your head. Like I described previously regarding "Stand at ease," paying attention to the speaker with your eyes is the backup to hearing with your ears. Aerobic listening means not just preventing your eyes from wandering off, but actually seeing *how* words are communicated by the speaker. Where in the conversation did they frown the most? When were they most excited? What were some of the big expressions (if any) during the conversation? All of this involves careful listening with our eyes. A fully-engaged listener notices the speaker's pauses, sees their chest rise and fall, even notices their blood pulsing in their neck. If so much of a conversation is *nonverbal*, then it can only be "heard" through sight. When I was a police officer, I used my eyes during interrogation almost more than I used my ears. You can *see* the truth or lies, not just hear them. Listening with your eyes is crucial.

I recently came across a news article entitled "Artificial Intelligence can diagnose PTSD by analyzing voices." It was referring to a 2019 study in *Depression and Anxiety* where "an artificial intelligence tool can distinguish—with 89 percent accuracy—between the voices of those with or without PTSD."[60] It goes on to say that more than 70% of adults

If so much of a conversation is nonverbal, then it can only be "heard" through sight. Listening with your eyes is crucial.

worldwide experience a traumatic event at some point in their lives and 12% of those struggle with PTSD because of those events.

The next time you're in a space filled with people, take a minute and look around you and think how 7 of every 10 have gone through some sort of trauma. And evidently the necessity of listening well is so prevalent that we are now creating AI to do it for us! Computers and software don't have ears, don't feel things, and yet they are able to "listen" with some 89% accuracy that someone is struggling. This startling fact ought to make us cringe a bit...How many of *us* can actually listen this well?

Listening well engages the body and helps others do the same, and as the next chapter will explore in some capacity, maintaining control over one's body in the present is absolutely key to dealing with trauma.

HOW AUTHENTIC LISTENING HELPED MY TRAUMA

When I returned home from Iraq after being away from my family for a solid 15 months, I remember standing in my living room, looking around, realizing it had been just a short six days from my last combat mission, and now I was home.

It was an indescribably weird experience. My whole life was *there*— gunshots, Humvees, endless sand. And now, in an instant, *I'm here*. Coffee shops, classes, and Nebraska grasslands. It was nothing short of a change of worlds. It obviously took some time to develop words to describe what had transpired throughout this whole ordeal, and because I didn't have the words, it became clear that things might easily come out in tears, depression, anxiety, or even isolation. This was uncharted territory.

The main problem at this point was that I had difficulty sleeping in my bed. It was twice as big as the one I had spent 15 months sleeping in. So, I ended up sleeping on the living room couch just to feel safe. I didn't know what was happening, and didn't have any words for it. I think all I said to my wife was, "I just need to sleep on the couch, honey; I don't know why, but I just do."

And Jodi listened. I was clearly changed, vulnerable, and a little frightened, but she listened with her whole body, listening to everything going on with *my* whole body. She didn't make me feel guilty when that would have been easy. Her bed had been empty for month after month—and now, even though I was home, it was *still* empty. But instead of pushing back, she loved and listened. She tucked me in, kissed me, and adjusted to this new and strange routine that lasted on and off for nearly three months.

Yes, it was strange. You would think that *this* would be the place I would be most secure—next to her in our own bedroom. But, looking back it was clear that survival instincts had taken over. I needed to be in a place where I had more control over my movements—where I was able to hit the ground quickly, or find the exit quickly, if something should happen. This wasn't contextually rational (who was going to hurt me, or what would really happen?), but that obviously didn't matter. I also slept less deeply on the couch so I could be more aware of sounds and movements; I was somehow aware that, being in bed with my wife, I ran the risk of getting *too* secure. I became captive to excessive alertness (or "hypervigilance").

Genuine listening is selfless—as we noted at the beginning of this chapter. And when later reflecting on this episode of our lives, Jodi did reveal that it was terribly difficult giving up our time together at night. In fact, she felt like I hadn't even returned from Iraq. (In some mental sense, I hadn't!) It wasn't a situation either of us wanted. But if I was going to improve at all, it required her to put aside her own needs for the time. She had to look past her own hurt to help heal mine. Genuine aerobic listening is really that in a nutshell: can you look past yourself, use all the muscles in your body to listen to the person communicating (verbally or nonverbally) about their trauma?

THE DIFFERENCE LISTENING CAN MAKE

I had been speaking on the Five Ls for about a month when I realized that I needed to make sure that I practiced genuine listening.

I was approached by a fellow veteran who had been struggling greatly with PTSD. She had been sexually assaulted while serving in the military. This is, of course, one of the great travesties in our military branches. I know of several friends whom I had the honor to serve with who are also victims of sexual assault or harassment within the military. This reflects the research, which shows that 1 in 4 women in the military have been sexually assaulted by someone in their chain of command (!).[61] The DoD SAPR annual report for 2016 and 2017 states that 14,900 members were sexually assaulted—8,600 women and 6,300 men. Most were sexually assaulted more than once, resulting in over 41,000 assaults in 2016 alone. It should sadden us that not only do military persons go through the trauma of combat where an enemy is on the prowl to destroy them, but that they must also endure violence from the people they should be able to trust.

Anyway, back to the conversation. The effects of the trauma were more than real: this individual did not feel safe leaving her apartment for about two weeks and wasn't able to complete necessary coursework. As she began to speak to me about her issues, it was clear that I needed to make a conscious decision to listen aerobically (to practice what I preach, so to speak). I squeezed everything out of my mind, all the stock "great advice," all of my own problems, all of the things I had to get done this day—everything. I pressed it out. I listened to her with my eyes, watched how each syllable and sentence made its way into the room, and let her thoughts and experiences enter my mind as fully as possible.

Soon enough, a critical threshold had been reached. Tears began streaming down her face, glistening in the light of the office, and her shoulders convulsed as she cried. I was feeling some of the pain she was experiencing. I never interrupted, and ensured that she owned this moment, because it was hers to own, and to share as she pleased. After this point, I just let time begin the kind of healing it can give before I said anything, and then sat with her in her pain as I continued to listen with my whole body. After another brief moment, I didn't launch into some long counseling session or provide a big list of "to-dos," but offered only a brief word, as nothing more was appropriate or necessary. She thanked me and left.

Later that day, a colleague of mine called to give me more of this particular veteran's story and to fill in some gaps. I listened to them with interest and concern. And then they remarked, "I wanted you to know that she came to my office right after she saw you, and she sat down and said, 'I don't know what just happened, but I feel like for the first time in my life, someone really heard me; they really listened to me'."

How many people had failed to listen and help this person heal? How many opportunities may have been missed due to someone else's busy schedule? I'll never know. But being present and empathetic in the moment made all the difference; it was a turning point for her.

And it was also a turning point for me. Because at that moment, my life changed. I realized the profound impact of listening we can all have.

CONCLUSION

"Now hear me out!"

We hear this phrase every day. And we hear it for good reasons: we *aren't* hearing people out. We're drowning in a sea of text, images and popular discourse.

People—all people, and not just those with trauma—are longing for someone to actually listen to them. Hopefully now, after reading this chapter, we might have the sensibilities and tools to be the kind of listener that we need to be for the people we love.

The question, once again, comes down to whether or not we will actually *love* the person or not. I really believe that unless you choose to love, then you will not listen. This is true for *any context* of communication—counseling, casual conversation, confession, even considering someone else's philosophical arguments written in a book. As renowned scholar Robert Wilken points out:

> The first task of a serious interpreter is to give oneself to the author. It was a point T. S. Eliot learned when studying Indian philosophy: 'You don't really criticize any author to whom you have never surrendered yourself...You have to give yourself up, and then recover yourself, and the third moment is having something to say, before you have wholly forgotten both surrender and recovery.' The student begins by putting himself or herself in the hands of a teacher who knows and loves the work...Love must precede argument.[62]

"Love must precede argument." Yes—and precede everything else!

I had the opportunity to present the Five Ls once to a group of university educators. One of them didn't see it this way. He insisted that he had listened to everything that I was saying, but said that he didn't know me well enough to love me, nor did he find it necessary to love in order to genuinely listen. I appreciated his honesty, but I just think he missed it: the choice to put someone ahead of yourself and understand what they're saying, for their sake, and entering into their world and letting it affect you, *is itself* an act of love. Yes, there are gradations and types of love. But generally speaking, it's not necessary to have prior knowledge of someone to love them. (When we're told to "love your neighbor as yourself," nobody reads this as "love only people you know well, because you can't love strangers.") So, call me stubborn, but I'm sticking with it: without love, you cannot truly listen.

Additionally, without listening you can't go further in your journey to do the next L, which is to *learn*.

QUESTIONS FOR REFLECTION

1. Have you ever felt truly heard? Reflect on that time and write down some memories of how you felt and how you knew you had been heard.
2. Have you tried to share something important with someone only to be brushed aside? Reflect on that time and write down your feelings and how you knew you were brushed aside.
3. When you're feeling hurt or anxious, what walls do you put up to avoid having to share anything to friends or family?
4. What's one or two things you wish people would "hear out"? Why so?
5. What are the biggest challenges for you, personally, to listening well?

3

LEARN

You live you learn, you love you learn
You cry you learn, you lose you learn
You bleed you learn, you scream you learn

ALANIS MORISETTE

Without the previous two Ls discussed in this book, it's impossible to *learn* anything of value. You have to decide that you will love, and then you really have to truly listen to the person reaching out to you. If you do this, then the next building block of helping a person who has gone through trauma can take shape. That block is *learning*.

Learn about what? First, we must learn about trauma—for your sake as an ally more than theirs as someone with PTSD. Why? Because it helps you put a context around what they say and do, so you don't end up taking it personally. It also helps us to avoid being captive to fear. Second, we must learn about our loved ones with PTSD—both their current experience and (as appropriate) their past experience. This second kind of learning is a *mutual* experience. It is learning *together*, and as you learn and reflect with them, they learn about themselves.

LEARNING ABOUT TRAUMA

On the one hand, modern Americans tend to be very independent people. And with the advent of the internet, many of us take on the role of self-created experts. We have the power of a quick Google search on our phones and feel empowered with "knowledge" to take on the world. Everyone is magically an all-knowing expert now.

On the other hand, modern people are also more dependent on specialists than ever before. There are medical programs dedicated to almost every part of the body. Most parents never talk to their kids about sex or racism or even the meaning of life because, well, that's what school teachers are for. We subcontract everything out. Hardly anyone knows how to start a fire or gather food in the woods, change the oil on their own car, or fix an electrical outlet in their own house. (Yep, we're kind of helpless sometimes!)

As we try to learn for the sake of our loved ones, there is yet again a balancing act: to be educated and informed, but not overconfident and arrogant—because part of the process of learning about our traumatized loved ones is to learn about trauma itself. Why? Because if we understand the mechanics of trauma, we realize how much those with PTSD just can't control it. Willpower isn't enough. Furthermore, understanding can dispel fear, because we fear what we do not understand.

Many children who have no exposure to dogs have a natural caution and anxiety about them and other animals. But once they understand what dogs are like—

Understanding can dispel fear, for we fear what we do not understand.

how they communicate, how they normally behave in different situations and why—their anxieties are relieved. Coming from rural America and the Great Plains, I know of some people who live in isolated areas who have a fear of dark-skinned people or people who speak another language. This is sometimes called "xenophobia," fear of outsiders and foreigners. Similarly, many in America are fearful of Muslims and their traditions because they simply don't understand them (this is "Islamophobia"). We often fear what we don't understand.

Similar to all of these situations is the fear of trauma and what it has done to our loved ones. Having a vivid PTSD episode for the first time is scary as hell. It's not just the trauma, it's the *awareness* of the trauma: *"What's happening to me?"* Or, *"What's happening to them?"* Dealing with PTSD—just like a person's unpredictable temper or manic episode—is all the more scary the less and less we understand.

The bad news is that the body, brain, and psychology of human beings is enormously complex and no research community is even close to mastering it all. The *good* news is, PTSD has been studied for over a half-century now, and we do have a basic understanding of its biological mechanics and can explain some of its most basic features. Science is often abused by corporate power and subject to change. But it can demystify things we experience and give us a more concrete orientation. So, what follows below is an ultra-condensed summary of those mechanics.

The mechanics and features of trauma and PTSD are ably summarized in Van der Kolk's influential work, *The Body Keeps the Score*. In the current scientific model, there are essentially three major components to the human brain that do different things and communicate with each other—the brain stem (controls essential functions we're not usually aware of), limbic system (fight/flight mechanisms, survival, appetites), and neocortex (higher thoughts, abstraction, judgments). Sensory input from our eyes, ears, and other sources generally goes from the "bottom up" instead of "top down"—that is, from the "primitive brain" (brain stem) to the "advanced brain" (neocortex).[63]

This is for survival reasons. We jump away from an object that looks like a snake, or pull our hand off a hot object before we are even able to *think* about it. And that's for a good reason: *this order of information transmission keeps us alive.*

Trauma, however, alters these survival and alarm systems. It establishes a pattern of reactiveness meant to keep us alive, but it gets in the way of our normal lives. We don't really need survival and energy hormones surging through our veins when we're going to bed on a normal evening, or increased blood pressure and heart-rates when driving a car on the freeway. But the connections have been made, and we respond accordingly, whether we like it or not.

PTSD is highly visceral—bodily. That's because the trauma happened *through* one's body. It's experienced through all our senses and our complex nervous system.

> Traumatic events push the nervous system outside its ability to regulate itself. For some, the system gets stuck in the "on" position, and the person is overstimulated and unable to calm. Anxiety, anger, restlessness, panic, and hyperactivity can all result when you stay in this ready-to-react mode. This physical state of hyperarousal is stressful for every system in the body. In other people, the nervous system is stuck in the "off" position, resulting in depression, disconnection, fatigue, and lethargy. People can alternate between these highs and lows.[64]

Any kind of healing and improvement, then, must involve *physical* practices as much as mental and spiritual ones.

> It is amazing how many psychological problems involve difficulties with sleep, appetite, touch, digestion, and arousal. Any effective treatment for trauma has to address these basic housekeeping functions of the body...Trauma affects the entire human organism—body, mind, and brain. In PTSD the body continues to defend against a threat that belongs to the past. Healing from PTSD means being able to terminate this continued stress mobilization and restore the entire organism to safety.[65]

Van der Kolk's general thesis, then, is that PTSD can be helpfully addressed from both the "bottom up" and "top down." "Bottom-up regulation involves recalibrating the automatic nervous system," which is "accessed through breath, movement, or touch." Top-down regulation is sort of the "mind over matter" approach—strengthening the capacity of your higher brain and mind to monitor your body and its sensations. "Mindfulness meditation and yoga can help with this."[66]

If this approach has any validity (and I don't see why it wouldn't), then we should think about treating and addressing trauma from a multi-faceted approach and not just a single approach. That's a subject that extends beyond this book, but hopefully it helps get you on some good footing, and explains how the wide-ranging themes of this book make sense given these mechanics of PTSD.

LEARNING ABOUT YOUR LOVED ONE: PART I

In addition to learning about trauma, we must develop strategies of how to effectively learn about our loved-one.

Helping our partners and friends tends to be challenging without knowing what they've been through. Trauma is often shrouded in darkness. It's omnipresent in a way, but continually unspoken at the same time. So, when those events come to light—sometimes in excruciating detail, this can be a turning point for the person and their relationships.[67] Some of the biggest acts of personal bravery and growth are when a person confronts the realities of the past, for example, being abused by a family member or of the present (coming out as non-heterosexual, as a member of a different religion, etc.). Some of the most positive, life-changing events in the lives of veterans is just talking about what they went through for the first time, whether to a friend or to a counselor. The pressure not to speak, after all, can be overwhelming. (What if my boss in the military finds out? What if my partner freaks out about what's happened in my life?)

This subject and process is fraught with risk, debate, and potential problems. Why? Precisely because conversations about the actual trauma are so sensitive. It is the locus and origin of the "stress" (the "S" in PTSD). Especially in the military community, there is enormous pressure just to keep quiet. Furthermore, you may be one of two kinds of people: fixers who want to get everything done and just force things ahead, or, the non-confrontational type who sweeps it under the rug—joining your loved one's silence and changing the subject anytime the events of the trauma come up.

Neither of these extremes are helpful. We need some kind of provisional guardrails for conversation and engagement. For starters, I want to dispel a potentially disruptive misunderstanding: *it is not absolutely necessary to know all the nitty-gritty details of a traumatic experience in order to help your loved one.*[68] Sometimes prying can cause deep distress to you both. In fact, even some professional therapies can re-traumatize the client and make things worse by digging too deep and too hard. So, I just want to underscore this point: genuine healing and progress *can* be made without full disclosure of what happened. Don't think that "he or she will never get better as long as they never tell me what happened." It's not that simple. *It's never right or helpful to compel your loved one to describe the events that are so traumatic to them.*[69] As we learned in the last chapter with that person who came into my office, what made that learning experience potentially healing and progressive in her journey was that it was her own. It was voluntary, and it happened when she was ready. We should *facilitate and catalyze* the process of opening up, unfolding, and unlocking, but never push it. (Loving involves patience.) "What is critical is that [the traumatized] learn to tolerate feeling what they feel and knowing what they know. This may take weeks or even years."[70]

How then, does one facilitate and catalyze a space for this kind of healing? Well, by *loving and listening*: being open, not shaming, or judging, making efforts to hear the speaker out on their own terms. When that happens, you probably won't even have to initiate a conversation to learn about what your friend or partner went through.

A friend of mine has a grandpa ("Lester") who was traumatized by the Korean War, and never spoke about it—until the last few years of his life. Details about the war unexpectedly came out at random points in conversation with his daughter and granddaughter. He was approaching 90 and had recently lost some of his closest friends, and death was on his mind, so he began opening up. On one occasion, Lester briefly recounted that an Army friend of his took his final patrol around the base just a day or two before flying back to the States, when he was unexpectedly killed. Lester was devastated and (evidently) never forgot it.

Why had he not said these things before? How could they be at the forefront of his mind over a half-century later? And, how can these memories be re-framed in a way that's more healing and less stressful?

This is where professional therapy can really help: it provides (or at least it *should* provide) a safe space to just unfold and recount things that have happened, and also develop new skills for re-wiring the body.

But most of the time, *you* are the one who will learn about these experiences. You will be the one entrusted with the intimacies of conversation. That's why it's important to be open (as much as feasible for yourself) to hear about whatever details your partner or loved one discloses. These are, after all, the vivid memories that regularly haunt them. And by learning about what specifically happened, you can develop specific strategies for mitigating triggers such as, not attending certain events, engaging certain activities, or using certain words. That's what we'll focus on in the next chapter. So, it's important to at least mentally prepare yourself for learning about disturbing scenes and events as much as this is possible. It probably won't be easy.

You can see, then, that this is a balancing act for both the traumatized and the learner:

a) Learning and sharing about the experience shouldn't be forced.

b) Yet, learning and sharing about the experience shouldn't be forced *away*.

c) The learner and listener must be active in listening and providing opportunities to hear whatever details are relevant to the experience.

d) Yet, the learner and listener must always consider when this might cease to be helpful to themselves and to the ones they're trying to help. (Sometimes the learner can be as easily triggered as those we're trying to help.)

It's an art and dance that requires adapting to each person and situation—and especially attending to each conversation.

If your partner is a closed book and you really want to inform yourself, it is not wrong or out of place to learn from others, and you shouldn't feel guilty for doing so. There are endless books and movies that do a fine job of capturing trauma and its effects, or just provide a factual account. (For example, Pulitzer-Prize winning journalist Chris Hedges wrote a popular book called *What Every Person Needs to Know About War*[71] that is specifically designed to inform—not sensationalize, downplay, or exaggerate—readers about the realities of war.)

All of this is to say that learning about the details of the traumatic experience may be a good and necessary part of the journey. Be prepared for it—prepared to listen, not react. Don't push it away if—or when—it comes. It is often an important step for the journey.

LEARNING ABOUT YOUR LOVED ONE: PART II

If learning about what happened is an important step of the journey, *how does one go about asking the right questions in the right way? How does one address our own fear in this process?* This is something a skilled therapist knows all about. But most days, you—friends and partners—are the ones who will hear these stories first.

The fact is this: once you establish Love (L1) and Listen (L2), we often don't know what to do from there. It's a weird experience: we long for people to open up to us, but when they do, we tend to retreat out of fear of what to say. For example, a friend of mine had a devastating miscarriage, and she shared some of the things that people said to her—people who undoubtedly cared. But they really didn't enter into her experience. They said things like, "you're young, you can have another." While this statement may be true, it was callous and dismissive.

...once you establish Love (L 1) and Listen (L2), we often don't know what to do from there. It's a weird experience: we long for people to open up to us, but when they do, we tend to retreat out of fear of what to say.

We've all been there. Someone shares something painful with us and we don't know how to respond, so we jump to platitudes, stock advice—anything to sort of get us out of the situation. Our fear can come from a place of caring and desire to protect someone from pain, but we fail because we haven't taken the time to genuinely listen and learn. We're afraid of uncertainty, or afraid of unintentionally hurting them, or even afraid of looking bad. But ultimately, we have to be willing to confront our own fears. It's not just about us and getting the right answer; it's about being there for the other person.

This means we have to ask the right questions, because asking the right questions makes all the difference. The right questions open new doors and possibilities. The wrong questions can be destructive. This obviously means it will take some effort at crafting and delivering good questions.

We must remember that *no question is neutral*. It always comes from a perspective, and with a certain tone. People use the phrase all the time, "...well, I was just asking." But they say that when they suspect that they've asked the wrong kind of question, or at least have already gotten some kind of reaction from it.

So, what's a good question? At the very least, good questions come from a place of *respect*. Respect for another person means knowing that:

1. You don't know what they experienced.
2. You don't know how to fix it.
3. You don't know how they will change and who they will be in the future.

Notice that all these things come from a position of *not* knowing—which makes sense if we're trying to learn. But this is an intentional not-knowing that continues through time. It's a *posture*, not a one-time goal, as if someday in the future we will have learned everything that there is to learn. Our whole attitude has to be centered on them and not ourselves (remember the first L). If it's not, questions can go south really quick. For example, I've been asked after returning from war, "How does it feel to kill someone?" and "So, how many people did you shoot?" These questions come from a position that's centered on the person asking it. It was for their own curiosity, and lacks respect for what I and others have gone through.

Centering our learning process on our loved ones also means we assume the posture of learner, not teacher. This also might seem obvious at first. But it is often tempting to take on the role of teacher or expert (or "Dad") in our conversations because *they* (our loved ones) are the ones needing help. This can compromise the mutuality of the relationship.

Other than a posture of respect and humility, good questions also distinguish between (a) where a person is and (b) what's happened to them or the problems they're currently facing. In other words, "the person is not the problem, the problem is the problem."[72] For a person who has experienced trauma, "the trauma" has a way of taking over that person's identity to the point where they can't recognize themselves anymore. They're no longer in touch with the hopes and dreams they have for themselves. Our questions can reinforce one of these directions over the other. We can continually frame the *person* with trauma as the problem, or we can frame *the trauma* as the problem.

> *..."the trauma" has a way of taking over that person's identity to the point where they can't recognize themselves anymore. They're no longer in touch with the hopes and dreams they have for themselves... We can continually frame the* person *with trauma as the problem, or we can frame the* trauma *as the problem.*

It's important, then, that our questions bear out this distinction. One way you can do this is asking about the different effects and influence of the *problem on them* instead of framing them as a problem. Instead of asking, "Why are you blowing up at me?", you can ask, "What effects do you think _____ has had on our relationship/on you?" This way of asking creates space for them to think about how they want to navigate the trauma, because it separates the two. This distinction also re-instates their agency so they can take responsibility for their actions. The problem isn't simply *them*. It's something distinct from their identity that they can choose to deal with.

Another line of inquiry you can use has to do with resurrecting and clarifying what's important to them in life. For example, you might ask, "In our talks, it seems like _____ is important to you. Is that true? Are there other times in your life where this value was really important to you? Can you share more about this with me?" This helps them see through the fog of trauma and experience themselves as someone who is capable of being who they want to be. Instead of someone who is stuck or trapped, they can see other options for themselves. This way, their imagination, desires and hopes are more easily rekindled.

Once they're able to see and experience that the problem is external to themselves and not simply them, and they begin to see new possibilities, you can then begin asking questions that re-establish their identity—their new or transformed identity. They may want to bring some of their "old self" into their life now, or make more dramatic changes. It may be a struggle for us if our loved ones want to discard parts of their old selves that we're attached to. But we have to respect this process of transformation. In the spirit of the Golden Rule, we respect the possibility of change for others as we would respect that possibility for ourselves.

Throughout this whole journey of learning and asking questions, it's important to remember:

1. *You don't have to solve it.* This reminds us to take it slow and relieve the weight on our shoulders. The reason why we make mistakes and say the wrong things is because of the *pressure* to fix things. But that pressure is manufactured and unnecessary. We mostly just need to be present.
2. *You can't take their pain away.* It's so difficult to watch someone we love suffer. You can relieve someone's suffering by walking alongside them, but you can't expect to just remove such powerful trauma on your own.
3. *You can still have a healing conversation without healing all at once.* A wound needs pressure to stop bleeding at some moments, but most of the time it needs lots of gentleness, patience, and regular checkups through time. It's OK to take lots of breaks, and it's OK to laugh about it. Just because a problem is serious doesn't mean you can't approach it with humor—especially when it's clear that the PTSD is the problem, not the person with PTSD.

CONCLUSION

Learning about trauma can help us orient to the changes in the mind and body of our loved one. Sometimes we need to address our own fears before entering into tough healing conversations with others. The process of redefining oneself after trauma can be lifelong, and you can be a powerful opener and support on this path your loved one is on. Hopefully this chapter has outlined some signposts to guide your journey.

QUESTIONS FOR REFLECTION

1. How can you open yourself up to learning more about those in your life who've experienced trauma?
2. What is your biggest fear in learning about your loved one's trauma?
3. Why do you think intimate conversation is both hazardous, difficult, and challenging on the one hand, but healing, bonding, and encouraging on the other?
4. What's the most healing question you've ever heard, and what made it so good? What's the most harmful question you've ever heard, and what made it so bad?
5. What do you think are obstacles to good communication with your loved one?

4

LESSEN

The crowds roll by and I keep falling in
Everyone's invincible, but it's just pretend
And we all freaked out, what a shame
When only tears know how to remind us we all break the same
We all break the same...

"Break the Same"
MUTEMATH

It was hot out that day.

The sun was beating down and the sounds of the crowd that surrounded me were both safe and yet unsettling. I sat watching people move to and fro, weaving in and out of conversation all without a care in the world. We were all sitting around in trusty lawn chairs eating the traditional American cuisine of burgers and hotdogs with ice cold sodas in hand. The church had some patriotic banners fliting on the fence close by. I found it odd that everyone appeared unaware of the busy movement going on around them—and all of the loud bangs that enveloped the air. The echoing cracks and booms seemed to roll off of the crowd as if they weren't even heard.

How can they do this?
How is it you're not flinching, and why aren't you looking around in
every direction trying to figure out what's up?
Perhaps, I thought, *I just need to get away from this and hit the mobile*
latrine in the church parking lot. Yes, that will do; I'll get my bearings
there while ridding myself of a few of these sodas at the same time...

It was Nebraska on July 4th, so it was a particularly dense and humid heat wave. I was sweating bullets, and while standing in that port-a-john, I began to feel transported...

To Iraq.

The sweltering heat, tight space, and familiar, dank smell of the latrine emanating from below was a familiar experience downrange in Iraq. And since the bathroom is often a place of pause and reflection, in my mind I began recalling all kinds of memories about this and that—but especially memories of wanting to be home and away from all this madness of war.

And then...

BANG! Pop! Pop! Pop!

My body dropped to the floor. I stopped breathing, and then began breathing rapidly. The heart inside my chest doubled its rate, pounding like a drum as fresh adrenaline coursed through my veins. My eyes flitted back and forth frantically, and I instinctively reached for my weapon...only to find that I didn't have one.

Where are the shots coming from? Where's the nearest defense? How long
should I stay here before running out for better cover? My mind raced through a series of options in a matter of seconds that seemed like an eternity. I had to survive whatever this was.

And then, moments later, it hit me.

I wasn't in Al Taqaddum.

I wasn't hearing small arms fire.

I wasn't even in danger.

I was in my own church parking lot, and Independence Day fireworks were being set off by kids from the youth ministry. Knowing this, however, obviously didn't prevent me from nearly melting down. My body was completely arrested; I was once again confronted with the fact that "When the alarm bell of the emotional brain keeps signaling that you are in danger, no amount of insight will silence it."[73]

After pulling myself back together and taking a few controlled breaths, I walked out cautiously. I remained on high alert even though I could see with my own eyes where I was and what was going on. It didn't matter. My brain and body had been trained over the course of 15 months to respond to (perceived) threats in a certain way. I walked across the lot and finally found Jodi. She was sitting and talking to friends. She looked up and knew right away that something wasn't right. She stood up, called for our kids, and politely excused us from the gathering.

Let's go home, babe.

In that moment, those were the most powerful words ever spoken to this broken soldier. It was as if storm clouds had cleared in my mind. My heart rate began to stabilize, and my breath returned to normal. I got in the car and we went home. And though that evening was not unicorns and rainbows (because the fireworks burst on), I was able to at least find solace in my sanctuary called home.

I survived the day.

THE TRIGGERS THAT AREN'T ON GUNS

It took me a long time to put words to what my wife did that day, but this reflection was part of the whole process, and it brings us to the fourth L: Lessen.

It's simple but important enough for this book to merit its own chapter. What Jodi did was *directly and strategically lessen the opportunity for further trauma*. She noticed my triggers (Learn) and used emotional intelligence and empathy (Love) and took me out of the situation (Lead, chapter 5). The more we can successfully perform this kind of mitigation, the greater chance we have in overcoming our trauma.

Here's a military-grade illustration. Let's say me and a buddy go out to have some cold ones. So we wander into a Marine bar and of course my buddy can't help himself, so he's yelling "Marines eat crayons!" and "You know what M.A.R.I.N.E. means, right? Muscles Are Required, Intelligence Non-Essential!" So, he gets into a bar fight with the crayon-eaters and…we both nearly die.

Here's the tough question: is it smart to bring him back to this place the next time we tie one on? Heck no! I'd obviously take him to a bar with Army folk so we can all *safely* make fun of the Marines *together*. (To all my Marine buddies, you know I had to!) Taking my buddy back to the Marine bar allows for further trauma to happen where taking that out of the equation does the opposite; it lessens the opportunity for further trauma.

Some of you are probably saying, "well that's easier said than done!" I get that. For some victims of trauma, the triggers are everywhere— including those places and situations that we would otherwise most enjoy (on the road, in bed, camping outside, etc.). Living each day can be like wading through an underwater mine field. It seems hopeless.

No matter the prevalence of triggers, there are still ways to lessen the opportunity for further trauma

But it isn't, because there's good news: *No matter the prevalence of triggers, there are still ways to lessen the opportunity for further trauma.*

We return to the power and simplicity of *embodied empathy*. After we have Listened and Learned about what our loved one went through, we can effectively develop practical routines and strategies to Lessen, which will create a greater tolerance and bandwidth to handle those tough situations.

For me, many of the triggering events are found on the highways and busy streets. Call it a special case of "road rage." When people are aggressive in their driving, it lights a small flame inside me that wants to grow and burn hotter and hotter. The first few times it happens in a commute, it rarely bothers me. But when these moments are compounded, it can reach critical mass. So? The shorter the commute, the less opportunity for further trauma to happen to me. That might complicate some scheduling issues, but often enough, it's a simple solution to keep things manageable.

What many people don't realize about trauma and its effects is that once you've experienced it to the point where it literally changes you, you're dealing with it physiologically whether you are aware of it or not.

> Because traumatized people often have trouble sensing what is going on in their bodies, they lack a nuanced response to frustration. They either react to stress by becoming "spaced out" or with excessive anger. Whatever their responses, they often can't tell what is upsetting them.[74]

In fact, "memory loss has been part of the criteria for PTSD since that diagnosis was first introduced."[75]

It's sometimes said that your body is putting up continuous walls to things that might retraumatize you. But every now and then, one of those walls gets penetrated by something and you snap back into survival mode. This happened to me when I was driving in Phoenix after a hike with Jodi.

We were heading out to find a place for brunch just after conquering a pretty serious trail—one that had almost killed the old out-of-shape-me a couple of years prior. I had lost a bunch of weight (about 70 lbs) and wanted to go back and see my improvements, and also prove to myself that I had come a long way and made real progress. And I had. (Got the Instagram photos to prove it, yo! Jodi took those photos on both occasions. She was happy to see that I wasn't close to heart failure the second time around!)

Anyway, we were going to a little breakfast joint that we love but in a different location than normal, so we needed to use the GPS to get there. As we were driving, I accidently cut someone off. This in turn caused the person I cut off to lose their cool and they began to drive in what appeared to me, as an aggressive manner—and laying on their horn all the while.

That sound triggered something in me that I hadn't felt in a long time. My heart began to race, my eyes narrowed, my teeth clinched and I zeroed in on the car. I chased the target down the road for some distance all while Jodi, helpless in the passenger seat, was yelling at me to stop. She yelled and pleaded, getting to the point of tears. The driver next to her wasn't acting anything like the person she was married to, or the one she had just enjoyed a celebratory hike with.

I finally came out of this monstrous episode and back to reality. I was angry, and yelled at Jodi to relax and to calm down and stop yelling at me. She sat there stunned and a bit scared. We drove in silence for a bit, and I pulled into a parking lot to gather myself before I spoke to her again. When I did, I lost it, and flat out bawled my eyes out. I rambled about how it made me feel.

And then it came to me: nearly every bit of combat trauma that I went through was from the inside of a vehicle. I realized this for the first time — thirteen years after combat. Every time I got in the front seat of my ASV in Iraq, it was full of trauma. Trauma from impending capture, violence, or death. Trauma from the random ear-deafening explosions, hailstorm of bullets, and other projectiles flying at highspeed in my direction. Trauma from dead bodies lying around in every direction, many of them an unrecognizable heap of body parts that were once animate people — someone's dad, mother, son, daughter, friend, partner. All of this time in the "normal world," I was removed from war — and yet, after more than a decade, my body and mind were still *living in* war.

LESSEN TO LIVE

I love my wife. After being scared to death, she let me weep and held me through that episode just like she had the countless others over the years. She regularly offers to take the wheel in order to lessen the opportunity for further trauma. She is now aware of what I went through and watches for the signs that one of my walls have been punctured. She checks in regularly to see how I'm doing and if I need any extra space as we traverse the streets of the Valley of the Sun together.

Your situation may not be as simple as getting a new driver for the person you care about. It might be dire—where you have to take decisive action to save a life, like getting someone into rehab. Many men and women who have suffered trauma do what they can to self-medicate. I know I have with alcohol over the years, and your friend or buddy may be going through the same thing. Feeling numb is better than feeling pain, right?

The use of those substances to cope with trauma will only introduce new traumas and will make it more likely that they experience the old trauma with greater intensity.

But here's the big problem with this wildly popular approach: It doesn't really work. In fact, it's actually counter-productive. *The use of those substances to cope with trauma will only introduce new traumas and will make it more likely that they experience the old trauma with greater intensity.*

And it is precisely in that space where suicide is prevalent for my brothers and sisters in arms. It's the hazy space somewhere between depressed and hopeless.

The best thing you can do to lessen further trauma for this loved one is to act positively: *get them the help they desperately need.* Get them to a professional tomorrow. Oh, I know: *but what if they don't want to? And what if the counselor is really lame?* I'm sorry to say that in these cases, it's the end of the line. It's that or death (or perhaps another 20 years under the spell of the bottle, which is a kind of death in and of itself).

So, let me be blunt: don't piss away the life of someone you love just because you are worried they will get mad at you for turning them in and getting them the help they need.[76] Desperation is desperation. (Do I really need to cite the suicide statistics again?) Besides, they will eventually get over it and end up being so grateful for your courage to do what they were unable to do in the moment. They may not see your love now, but they will later.

It's probably obvious to you by now that Lessening stands on top the other Ls that precede it. The greatest, of course, is Love. If you don't love, how can you find yourself caring so much for others? I am reminded of a severe lack of love and empathy having written this during the height of the COVID–19 pandemic. At the start of 2021 we were reeling from the loss of over 350,000 Americans and over two million globally—and still, the U.S. President and administration (2016-2020) continued to downplay the severity of it all—and publicly bully citizens just for wearing masks. Many of the President's words were laced with explicitly anti-empathetic discourse even as he and those in his inner circle almost died from the virus. This kind of behavior is more likely to *induce and fertilize trauma,* not mitigate it. Nobody needs that.

If we are to help our loved ones who are walking through and out of trauma at this very moment, we must do the right thing in showing empathy so we minimize the chances that they will be harmed by further traumatizing them.

CREATING A SAFE AND STABILIZING ENVIRONMENT

A couple of evenings ago, Jodi and I took the opportunity to set down and talk with our host daughter from India, Yestina. It was about six months ago now (in the midst of the pandemic) that she lost first her father to the virus and a week later her grandmother. Both her mother and brother had also tested positive as well.

Yestina found herself thousands of miles away from home when the news of her father's passing came to her. She and her younger brother had been working tirelessly to get him in the hospital. They reasoned that his symptoms were COVID-related but in India at the time, he could not be admitted to the hospital without a positive test. It was nearly impossible to get a test, but through some connections they were finally able to get one.

Upon receiving a positive result, he was admitted to the hospital and placed on a ventilator, only to succumb to the virus just moments later. The news was devastating. Then, a week later, word came that her grandmother also passed.

As you can imagine, the entire situation was traumatizing.

Unexpectedly losing a parent in your 20's is bad enough, but how much worse when you're thousands of miles away and unable to be there. (No flights from the U.S. were allowed to travel anywhere in the world at the time.) Her father was buried at a social-distanced funeral where her mother and brother could only watch from a vehicle. Yestina wasn't able to go home to say her goodbyes at all. Jodi and I were obviously here for her, but our help was limited.

Time sometimes does begin to heal wounds. But some of them are so deep that time stands still. On one particular evening, we sat down with Yestina to recuperate and talk. She discussed how we and her friends allowed her to cope with the loss simply by providing an environment with various possibilities for things to do. "It has been so nice," she said, "to be able to just step outside and hike or go for walks and watch sunrises and sunsets" to help get her mind off of her losses. Jodi and I had been thinking about anything we could do to help this grief-stricken soul, so when I heard this, I thought, *There it is*. Here is a clear way to lessen trauma for this person—and maybe a way for everyone.

Spaces and places to get your mind off of things are sort of like Band-Aids. They slow the bleeding to allow for your body to begin the long-term healing process. They aren't permanent fixes, but safe places along the path. And when many of these moments become a regular part of a traumatized person's life, they can have a stabilizing effect.

NATURE'S BALM IS NATURE ITSELF

For thousands of years, nature in particular has played a profound role in providing a sense of place, of grounding,[77] of something solid and firm for human life. It is among the trees and rivers and mountains and animals and plants and deserts and meadows where people have most often felt fully alive. Nobody writes awe-inspiring poetry about laboring in the dark coal mines or going up and down the elevators of a high-rise. But caving and climbing granite cliffs, swimming under water along the shores of a mountain lake with the fish to your right and rays of sun on the moss to your left, and laying down for sleep in a hammock to the pitter-patter and gentle rumbles of a sweet-smelling summer rain storm, that's another story.

> When I would re-create myself, I seek the darkest wood, the thickest and most interminable and to the citizen, most dismal, swamp. I enter as a sacred place, a *Sanctum sanctorum*. There is the strength, the marrow, of Nature. (Henry David Thoreau, *Walking*, 1851)[78]

> The deeper we look into nature, the more we recognize that it is full of life, and the more profoundly we know that all life is a secret and that we are united with all life that is in nature. [People] can no longer live [their lives for themselves] alone. We realize that all life is valuable and that we are united to all this life. From this knowledge comes our spiritual relationship with the universe. (Albert Schweitzer, 1875-1965)[79]

> The best remedy for those who are afraid, lonely or unhappy is to go outside, somewhere where they can be quiet, alone with the heavens, nature and God. Because only then does one feel that all is as it should be and that God wishes to see people happy, amidst the simple beauty of nature. As long as this exists, and it certainly always will, I know that then there will always be comfort for every sorrow, whatever the circumstances may be. And I firmly believe that nature brings solace in all troubles. (*Diary of Anne Frank*, February 23, 1944)

I won't even mention the amazing poetry of Emily Brontë, Ralph Waldo Emerson, or the Hebrew wisdom literature on this subject.[80] But hopefully the point is clear: nature is larger than life, we as human beings are nature aware of itself, and this connection largely determines the health of our own spirit.

This is more than a romantic theory. It's been verified by contemporary research.

> Women dealing with the trauma from breast cancer are able to focus better when they spend time in Nature. Depressed people who stroll in green places have significantly better moods than those who walk city streets. Recently, Gregory Bratman and his Stanford colleagues have shown that city dwellers who walk in Nature for only ninety minutes

decrease activity in the subgenual prefrontal cortex, an area of the brain associated with morbid rumination, the repetitive, unproductive chewing over of negative thoughts about our lives and ourselves— exactly the kind of self-defeating mental activity that hobbles the brains of traumatized and depressed people...Research in England shows that people living among farms, fields, and meadows are less stressed and depressed, and they live longer than those in less green areas...In Japan, research on... "forest bathing," has shown the therapeutic power of walking in the woods, enjoying the sights, and breathing in air perfumed by leaves and bark with medicinal properties.[81]

Is it any wonder, then, that "the first man to walk the entire Appalachian Trail from Georgia to Maine was a World War II veteran named Earl Shaffer, who had decided to 'walk the army out of my system, both mentally and physically'"[82]? It isn't for me!

As a resource for trauma recovery, grounding can help you reclaim a sense of safety, feel rooted in the present moment, and strengthen your resilience.[83]

And here's something else to think about: what if we could create a *micro*cosmos of the cosmos, just shrink down the world and calming experience of nature into the size of, say, a human being? Wouldn't that be incredible?

That's exactly my point: *you and I* can join the wilderness as a sort of balm or Band-Aid for someone we love. We don't have be the professional counselor or critical incident debriefer. But we can be that essential, temporary cover for someone going through the healing process, the person that people find restful and restorative like a walk in the woods or along an ocean shore.

I look forward to the day when Yestina can walk out of her trauma—just as I do so many of my fellow veterans who are still struggling with war long after hanging up their uniform.

QUESTIONS FOR REFLECTION

1. Do you have some "Band-Aids" in your life? What are some things you can do to help ease your own pain or the pain of your loved one going through trauma?

2. Are you purposeful about steering clear of things that cause you further trauma, or do you knowingly put yourself in situations that can cause you to experience trauma because you think you aren't worth saving?

3. Is nature-walking or time outdoors a part of your routine? What practical steps can you take to ensure you breathe good air, sink your toes into some grass, sand, or river pebbles, and feel part of something vast and immense?

5

LEAD

And while devotion to principle or courage of conviction, perseverance and patience, and self-control are the predominating requisites of true leadership, over and above them all—embodying the truest leadership— is a deep and abiding love for humanity.

IDA B. WELLS

What exactly is great leadership?

I've learned from my graduate work in Sociology at Arizona State University that most people see leadership as a list of particular characteristics to be agreed upon. For instance, when a group of other graduate students put together the important leadership characteristics for a class project, they arrived at integrity, authenticity, mindfulness, flexibility, humility, inclusivity, a good listener, and empathetic. You might agree with them that these are important when it comes to leadership, as I do.

But as I compiled all of these characteristics into a graph, I found myself having different thoughts. Whereas most others seem to think of leadership primarily in corporate terms (like what makes a good CEO), I was thinking about leadership in a combat situation. Don't get me wrong; leading in combat needs to have the kinds of character traits mentioned above, and there's nothing wrong with corporate/organizational leadership in principle. But the fact is, there's just more to it when lives are on the line. The dynamics change, and the consequences are always bigger. So, grant me a few more pages of your time, and I'll explain what I mean—and how these specifics immediately apply to our leadership decisions regarding the traumatized.

WHEN THE BOMBS ARE REAL

It was a cool October night in the desert of Iraq.

Our team was on our first mission all by ourselves. We had just completed three missions with the unit we were replacing as convoy security. Saddam Hussein had just been hung for his war crimes in a suburb of Baghdad, and the Islamic holiday of Ramadan was upon us. I had been given the distinct (and scary) honor of being the truck commander for what we called the Rat Truck (or just "Rat"). Rat would lead "outside the wire" (beyond the confines of the base) and would travel anywhere from 500-1000 meters ahead of the rest of the convoy. I was given that job by my platoon sergeant who we called "Gunny." Gunny and I had come up in the ranks together and had been part of Charlie Battery (an artillery unit) back in the day. We were "cannon cockers;" we hailed from the artillery so we had been part of combat arms together.

All of this is significant for our story because most of the young soldiers in our platoon were combat service and support and had never really been trained at any level of sophistication about combat arms, so we had some catching up to do. We faced a very seasoned and formidable enemy.

I'll never forget the day Gunny gave me the job.

"You're a cop in the civilian world, right Preacher?" ("Preacher" at the time was not an occupational title I held, but a nickname I earned for being prayerful and passing out bibles stateside).
"Yes, Gunny. Why?"

"You must be brave do to that—and I need someone brave to lead us out in the Rat truck."

I was honored...but also terrified. My job was to travel out in front of the convoy with my driver and gunner and find IED's, or insurgents, or both, and then confront them—either by getting blown up so no one else would, or finding them and engaging them until reinforcements arrived. You may have heard the term frontline of battle. Well, this was about as frontline as you could get for a traveling convoy! It was *high*-risk.

I took what little knowledge I had and joined it with the "knowledge" I gained from just three missions with the unit we were replacing, and we left the FOB (Foreword Operating Base) on one fateful night in October. I say "knowledge" not as a dig against the unit we replaced (they were some brave men and women, no doubt), but simply to indicate that we just didn't really know the tactics of our enemy past a certain point. I can still quote to you what I learned:

1. Go fast enough that if you get hit by an IED, it might not kill you.
2. If you see something that looks fishy, it probably is, so don't run over it.
3. Make sure to radio behind you telling everybody what looks fishy.

Sounds like great advice really.
Well, it ended up being not such good advice after all.
This particular night we were heading to Al Assad and were protecting the convoy as we would for about another 100 missions. We passed our check point at pancake village, just outside Camp Al Taqqadum. (Pancake village was given its name after being flattened during Operation Iraqi Freedom.) We received a good copy and rolled off of ASR (Alternate Supply Route) Fiesta onto a different route called ASR Lemon. It was dark since we did most of our missions at night; our superior equipment for nighttime operations gave us an advantage over any insurgency in the Anbar province, or so we thought.

Speaking of the Anbar province, there was great optimism around our camp that we had essentially driven out the insurgency from there towards Baghdad, so we didn't have to worry so much about anything close to our own FOB. Turning onto ASR Lemon after a whole *three* missions worth of training, I felt fairly confident in my ability to lead my squad on this mission in the Rat truck.

My driver, gunner, and I had been together now for a couple of months and had become close. We were true comrades and partners in arms. To this day, I would give my life for them, no questions asked, even if what happened next may have splintered that a bit.

We were rolling along the road, and I was sitting in front of the ASV (Armored Service Vehicle) staring intently out the windshield for anything suspicious. Then, I saw what I knew to be an MRE (Meal Ready to Eat) bag in the middle of the road. We had learned in our training on IED's that the insurgency had been using our trash to blow us up. They were hiding detonators in various containers and bags, and we would drive over it not suspecting anything, but then once the pressure plate was pressed, it would detonate the explosive and destroy whatever drove over it. It was unusually effective in combatting a superior army like that of the U.S. We were moving at a pretty good clip, because apart from that bag, I couldn't see any wires or anything else unusual. (*Rule one: Drive fast in case you hit an IED because then maybe it won't' kill you.* Check!). So, I tell my driver, "Don't run it over!" (*Rule 2: If something looks fishy is probably is so don't run it over.* Check!) Knowing that it looked pretty fishy, I followed the third rule: I made the call back to the Lead gun truck, second in line in our convoy, which was about 1,000 meters behind us.

I can remember what I said.

"Lead! Lead! This is Rat. Be advised, MRE bag in the middle of the road. Looks fishy. You may want to check it out."

What I heard in response is as vivid now as it was then, forever etched into my consciousness:

That's a good copy Rat, we'll take a loo…

An immense *KABOOOOM!* abruptly cut off his voice. We could feel the explosion in our chests nearly a klick away.[84] All gun trucks responded on the radio, "IED Det! IED Det!" (meaning IED detonation). With those key words reverberating over the speakers, it was clear what we needed to do. Some of us would take up defensive positions in case any hostiles were ready to pounce, while others would take up the job of recovery operations and life-saving actions.

We all did what were trained to do, but the "drive fast" rule proved wrong. The explosion had already taken its toll. Three of our troops were severely injured, including a good friend who, to this day, is living with traumatic brain injury.

What does this story have to do with genuine leadership? Well, it taught me something about leadership that I didn't find in my graduate coursework, and that's this: *Good leaders take responsibility for both the good and bad things that happen, and great leaders bring order to chaos.*

I came to realize this because I was initially (and perhaps even today in a sense) held responsible for our first casualties of war for our unit. My mishandling of that destructive IED caused our friends to get blown up.

> *Good leaders take responsibility for both the good and bad things that happen, and great leaders bring order to chaos.*

I still hold this burden close to my heart even today. I felt that night that everyone hated me or had abandoned me, but good leaders allow for that higher accountability to happen so their troops can lighten any guilt they may have—so that they push on. It's a war thing. I don't think most people would understand it.[85] I liken it a bit to what Simon Sinek speaks about in how leaders eat last. It is true military leaders are trained to eat after their troops in the chow line, but it goes deeper than that. I think lightening of responsibility should go first to those you are leading so that they are able to function. Leaders take on a heavier load for the good of the team.

Looking back, I know that what I learned that night on that dark, chaotic Iraqi road was invaluable for the rest of the year we spent there. I learned that, contrary to the standard training recommendations, you *don't* go fast, but slow, so you can see what is in front of you and don't run over anything *and* have a chance to call it out for everyone else's sake. This is bringing order to chaos, sanity and calm to unbelievably stressful situations where everyone is potentially a split-second away from sudden death. I learned that if something is fishy looking, then you better not just pass it by and let your buddies blow up behind you. This again, is bringing another bit of order to chaos.

What does this have to do with the Five Ls? It's simple: your loved ones who are struggling right now with PTSD are living in a world of chaos. As we learned earlier, people in this condition are (or at least chunks of their body and brain are) living in that historic event of trauma. For me, that means my mental alarm system and body got stuck in a sort of permanent state, always driving that Rat truck, paranoid about explosives in front of the car.

The way I used to handle stressors in life is now disordered. It's chaotic. The way I think I should act or how my body should react are not the "normal" way anymore. After (Post) my trauma event (Traumatic), handling stress (Stress) is chaotic (Disorder). So, if you *Love* someone, and *Listen* to them in an aerobic way, and *Learn* where their trauma comes from, and you do what you can to *Lessen* further trauma, you are already doing the last L. You are that person in the middle of their chaos that is bringing order. You are the leader that they are looking for. You don't have to have all the answers. You don't have to portray all of the aforementioned leadership characteristics. But what you need to do is be willing to reach down into the dark and chaotic space your loved one is living in and do what you can to pull them back into the light.

Leaders are sometimes said to be people who "take the initiative," and that's right. Whether anyone likes it or not, people like me who have struggled with and are still struggling with PTSD are looking for someone like you to do just that. We are hurting at a level that we can't deal with on our own. We need a "battle buddy" if you will. We need someone to provide practical help as we work our way through the trauma that has happened.

The Five Ls

LEADERSHIP IN THE WILDERNESS

During a recent trip to the Mogollon Rim outside of Pine, Arizona, I was once again reminded of the necessity of great leadership. As a part of the Huts for Vets Wilderness Healing team, we ventured on a difficult 13.5-mile hike along the beautiful Geronimo Trail. We spent three days in the wilderness with veterans who have been struggling to make sense of things post-war or post-trauma of some kind. I was asked back for this third trip (the other two being in the majestic Rockies near Aspen, Colorado) to be a leader and facilitator of our readings, and a "guide" towards some sort of relief. The head honcho you already heard from in the foreword to this this book, Paul Andersen. I have watched this man (who is not a veteran by the way) launch young men and women into this incredible healing journey, and I have always been struck by the way that he leads.

One of the readings along the trail that help veterans begin to open up is a reading from Aldo Leopold called "Thinking like the Mountain." Here's an excerpt:

> A deep chesty bawl echoes from rimrock to rimrock, rolls down the mountain, and fades into the far blackness of the night. It is an outburst of wild defiant sorrow, and of contempt for all the adversities of the world. Every living thing (and perhaps many a dead one as well) pays heed to that call. To the deer it is a reminder of the way of all flesh, to the pine a forecast of midnight scuffles and of blood upon the snow, to the coyote a promise of gleanings to come, to the cowman a threat of red ink at the bank, to the hunter a challenge of fang against bullet. Yet behind these obvious and immediate hopes and fears there lies a deeper meaning, known only to the mountain itself. Only the mountain has lived long enough to listen objectively to the howl of a wolf.[86]

Only the mountain has lived long enough to listen objectively to the howl of the wolf. This statement hangs suspended in my mind as I think back about our recent trip. It makes me ponder how leading well takes time. I think fondly of Paul, and how, over decades of knowing the mountain, he understands those who venture into the mountain wilderness to find the healing they deeply long for. In fact, I made a statement about Paul himself during our trip, and I hope he reads this with great fondness as I share it here with you:

> The mountain may indeed listen to the howl of the wolf,
> but Paul is a man who truly embodies the mountain.

Leading so often in our culture today is done by people who have not had the time to marinate their understanding. They are leading like they were just popped out of the microwave. They've barely graduated college and are already touting themselves as experts, consultants, and life coaches. What this world and your loved ones need is someone leading from living what I call a *slow-cooked life*.

Back when my kids were young, on Sunday mornings I used to put a roast in the oven before church. I would slice an onion in half and place it over the roast, along with generous salt and pepper. Along the sides of the Dutch oven, I would carefully place carrots and potatoes to be softened for lunch upon our return home. Placing it in the oven, I knew that when we opened the backdoor, the aroma of that roast, along with the vegetables and spices, would waft out to greet us. This smell is what I call "Sunday morning."

...And you're wondering at this point, *what does that have to do with leadership?*

In a word, *genuine leadership requires seasons of life, a little spice, and marination, or it's not going to smell good*. What I've come to learn over my years, and watching a man like Paul, is that leading comes from a place of allowing yourself to take the time needed to do it well—to allow for others to come close to you in the slow cooker of life, for you to season their lives as they season yours. Leadership should be slow-cooked (or a "patient ferment," to borrow from one author)[87] to allow for you to smell like Sunday morning to someone in need. When they know you are "fully-cooked and seasoned well," it will be easier for them to receive your leadership. They will, in fact, smell that wafting from the kitchen and come to you with less defenses. They will know instinctively that they can follow you. This type of leadership, the slow-cooked kind, allows the follower to trust and be at ease, even over the rocky and difficult hikes in life.

Perhaps you think this doesn't apply to you because you don't have enough gray hair. But the beauty of the slow-cooked life is that even the young can smell like Sunday morning. Yes, you have to live in order to help others live. But after a certain point, age is not a reliable indicator for either maturity or immaturity. (Some folks never collect the right ingredients for their roast, and others never get it in the oven until halfway through life.) As I mentioned before, if you simply take your time getting to know yourself and those around you, you can truly grow. Don't jump to conclusions about things, but instead, allow your feelings to make themselves known. Live in the moment, breathe deeply before acting. Take walks, allow your past to transmit wisdom to your soul. We all have a history, no matter our age, so allow it to speak to you in the present.

I think for me, the slow-cooked life is about pacing myself. I remember when I was in high school (back when dinosaurs roamed the earth), and I was a shotput and discus thrower on the track team. Our coach told us on our way to a meet that all weight throwers would have to enter a running event. Now, I have never been fleet of foot, so this was not something I was looking forward to. I kicked around the different events in my head and decided to sign up for the 400-yard dash. In my mind, "dash" meant something for sure, and I figured I would be able to sprint my way to a good showing. There I was for my first and only time in the starting blocks, then the gun! I took off like a flash (well, at least I felt that way). I rounded the first corner, and to my surprise, I was out in the lead. I pressed on, and we were at around 200 yards when I looked over my shoulder to see that I was still leading. I couldn't believe it! But then it happened. I ran out of gas. It was like my legs were moving, but I wasn't getting anywhere. Everyone passed me by, and in the end, I was dead last in my heat by a long shot!

I have reflected on this many times over the years because it was a moment where I was way out of my comfort zone and truly vulnerable. I have never enjoyed losing anyway, but this loss was not a close call, it was a flat-out pummeling. The loss and race itself gave me perspective though.

I should have paced myself. Instead of jumping out to some crazy lead in the first 200, I could have started slower. I should have started at a pace I could maintain the entire race. I reasoned it would take some practice, but I know now that pace and rhythm are essential to track athletes and life in general. It's the same with living the slow-cooked life: learn from your mistakes and take into account the pace and rhythms of life.

I challenge you today, as you decide to help a loved one through trauma, that you take a close look at yourself. Will you continue to live in such a way that you smell like Sunday morning? Can you take the time necessary to lead well? I hope so. People could be counting on you to one day lead them out of the dark and into the light.

LEADERSHIP AND POST-TRAUMATIC GROWTH

At the end of the day, trauma is not solely a bad thing that hurts and damages. The challenges of trauma can function as a catalyst for building ourselves—our person, our character, our bodies—into something better than if these events never happened. I know this might sound like a wild idea to some (like the idea that good can come from evil), but it's kind of like reflecting on young, romantic breakups: they're the worst thing in the world, but some of them are also the best thing that could have happened to us.[88] The result? Growth.

Post-traumatic Growth (PTG) simply suggests that we can become more resilient people as a result of confronting and properly handling our PTSD.

> You can foster resilience by focusing your attention to that which supports your physical, mental, emotional, social, and spiritual well-being (McGonigal, 2015). You can build *physical* resilience by getting enough exercise, eating a healthy diet, and attending to the impact that traumatic life events have had on your body. You can build *mental resilience* by adopting a mindset that recognizes your capacity to grow, even through challenges. You can build *emotional resilience* by processing traumatic events in therapy and through personal journaling. You can build *social resilience* by staying connected to other people instead of

isolating. You can build *spiritual resilience* by attending to a deeper sense of personal meaning and purpose. Most importantly, you can support your resilience with the belief that your choices and behaviors make a difference in the outcome of your life. This gives you the confidence that you are in charge of actively creating opportunities that allow you to overcome barriers in your life.[89]

This last aspect is important, because trauma is all about things happening to a person that are out of their control. This is why many of the effects of trauma are often centered around *establishing* control (like me sleeping on the couch to make sure I could move quick). As we discussed at the end of chapter three, when we come to see that our choices do matter, that we are agents in the world with real power, life becomes less chaotic around us.

> Resilience is both a process and an outcome. As a process, resilience involves engaging in behaviors that support your well-being each and every day…As an outcome, resilience involves experiencing yourself as capable of handling life's challenges and the choices you've made that determine the outcome of your life. You are able to look at your most difficult events and say, "This happened to me—and it is over now." Turning toward pain builds character. It provides you with an opportunity to realize that you are stronger than you previously believed…As you feel stronger, you are more likely to see yourself as able to bring your gifts and contributions to the world.[90]

At first, my traumas never appeared to have any good or enduring aspects to them. Trauma from my childhood or time as a police officer—and certainly my trauma from war—all seemed irreparable. But because people in my life took the time to lead me well, I was eventually able to see how coming through those traumas created a stronger sense of empathy for others around me. I have always felt a sense of empathy for people. But what I have gone through brought me to a place where their trauma is actually more real to me. I am able to help them at a greater depth than before because their experience is also mine. It took others who I leaned on, those who have led, to show me how I had grown.

Growth is an odd thing in that (unless it is your weight after Thanksgiving turkey) you often don't notice it at first, and you need people to point it out. So, it's important to take the time to tell your loved ones the growth you see in them. They may be focusing only on their trauma and unable to recognize their growth in other areas. I hope you will be the leader in your loved one's life that pays attention enough to see the positives in their life.

QUESTIONS FOR REFLECTION

1. Write down what you think makes a good leader and reflect on whether or not you embody those characteristics.
2. Who in your life was or is a great leader? What about them do you admire?
3. Has your idea of leadership changed at all since reading this chapter? If so, how?
4. Have you seen Post-traumatic Growth in you or your loved one? What does that look like?

CONCLUDING REFLECTIONS

Life is a hard battle anyway. If we laugh and sing a little as we fight the good fight of freedom, it makes it all go easier.
I will not allow my life's light to be determined by the darkness around me.

SOJOURNER TRUTH

The advantage of a book based on an acronym is that it's easy to memorize and markets itself pretty well. The disadvantage is that not everything fits. So, I want to tie up a few loose ends real briefly before bringing this whole project to a close. In doing so, I want to talk more directly to those who are struggling.

A DOSE OF HOPE GOES A LONG WAY

Hope is the thing with feathers that perches in the soul and sings the tune without the words and never stops at all.
— EMILY DICKENSON

I hope this book has given you *hope*. Why? Because without hope, there is no reason to live. But with hope, well, the benefits are numerous and immediate:

Hope significantly improves performance in life, as well as recovery from illness. Children and young people who are hopeful are far more likely to focus on success rather than being preoccupied with failure; they do better academically and athletically. Students who are more hopeful are less likely to see poor grades as a sign of personal inadequacy...Hopeful adults are more flexible, committed, and imaginative; they function better at work. Hopeful older adults are far less reactive to stressful events. Hope decreases suffering from chronic pain and extends our survival from life-threatening illnesses like cancer. People who are more hopeful live longer.[91]

Like so many things in life, there is a "life-balance" to achieve. Excessive optimism can terminate in mass delusion, while extreme cynicism is toxic to everything and everyone. I know people who listen to the same radio and TV shows every day, and everything is doom and gloom when you talk to them. Other people seem perpetually happy, like they swallowed the warmth of the sun, and I can't even imagine what it would be like to see them cry. There's plenty of reasons to be cynical in this world—and plenty of reasons to be optimistic.

Many of our perceptions are shaped by personality and things we don't necessarily change. But our perceptions are also constructed by society, the world around us, and the world created for us in media for our mass "consumption." My conclusion is this: it's important to take each episode of life with a dose of both realism and hope, but to ultimately lean in the optimistic direction (as hard as that is sometimes).[92]

...it's important to take each episode of life with a dose of both realism and hope, but to ultimately lean in the optimistic direction (as hard as that is sometimes).

We have to be informed about the suffering of others—the children needlessly drone-bombed overseas, the famines created by civil war, the vulnerable communities in our cities that struggle to survive. We can't help people and problems if we don't know they exist. But we must protect our eyes and ears to those toxic levels of negativity that seep into our bones and make us a hopeless crank. These thresholds are different for each person, so I can't tell you want kind of limits to establish. (For example, a friend of mine—the person on this book cover, in fact—had to stop reading about the melting of polar ice-caps because it just creates too much anxiety.) But think about it and take action: if you're a cynical person, are you feeding yourself too much negative information? Plug-in to podcasts, music, blogs, and even new friends, that pull you in a more optimistic direction. If you're an overly optimistic person who hates conflict, then challenge yourself to *really hear* the voice of the suffering by plugging into not popular doomsdayers (remember: *lean in the optimistic direction*), but people and media and things that at least can break through your bubble and remind you that evil still exists in this world. Because "injustice anywhere is a threat to justice everywhere" (Martin Luther King Jr.). We have work to do.

We're all pulled in so many directions each day. I know I am. One day, everything seems hopeless, and I don't know why I'm even trying to write this book. On other days, I have full conviction that injustice and suffering and death won't have the last word in this universe, and that we were made to attain peace, freedom, justice, and wholeness.

I lean in this optimistic direction, and I think that we all know in our heart of hearts that not only does this hopeful outlook keep us alive, but it's better for us, and that we're made for a better future.

OUR FURRY FRIENDS MATTER

This one is more simple: pets (properly trained and maintained) are a profound source of comfort and stress-relief.

> Several studies on healthy adults and those with hypertension have demonstrated that brief sessions with animals can decrease blood pressure. One small study published in the *Journal of Psychosomatic Research* showed that this positive change was accompanied by decreases in the stress hormone cortisol, along with increases in mood-elevating beta endorphin, energizing dopamine, and oxytocin, the hormone responsible for bonding...Erika Friedmann and her colleagues published a particularly dramatic study of successful animal therapy. Pet-owning people who had been hospitalized with heart attacks for...heart-related pain had significantly greater one-year survival rates than petless patients...

Trauma may make us withdrawn, fearful, and suspicious. Our connection with animals, our sense of being known and accepted by them, and of caring for them, can be a living bridge bringing us back to caring for and connecting with other people.[93]

I've always had a dog in my adult life, and I can testify to these findings by personal experience. You can therefore imagine my grief as I type these words.

The past two weeks have been a little tough here on the home front. Jodi and I lost both of our best friends. Our dog Annie went "over the rainbow," as it were. She was a family pet her whole life, which spanned an incredible 16 years and 6 months. Nessie followed suit two weeks later after a good life with us for over 11 years. Though Annie and Nessie were never trained to be (nor would claim to be if they could speak), they were truly an emotional support while I healed from war. They were there for me in a way that I have only recently understood.

The odd thing about our dogs, in a way, is that *they* did all of the Ls as well. I know I spent time sharing my struggles with them. They listened to me intently. They learned what they could from my emotions and actions, and maybe even tempered their behavior to be closer to me in times of anguish. They kept me happier than I might have been otherwise, which probably lessened further trauma for me. Finally, in the way only a dog can do, they led me on walks, led me outside for things, led me away from detrimental behaviors by simply being a part of my life. On many occasions during those first few months after being home, Annie would sleep with me on the couch instead of in bed where she normally slept. It was like she knew and wanted to be close to me. I don't claim to know anything about the mind of a dog, but I can say that Annie and Nessie were truly "a man's best friend" during my journey to heal from trauma.

CONCLUDING REFLECTIONS

EAT HEALTHY AND EXERCISE
(Shocking, right?)

Along with the true love of a pet, a few other things I have found that have facilitated relief and healing are eating healthy and getting in shape. I know that's not breaking news to you. And it's not new scientifically "Study after study has shown that a variety of whole foods diets, can reverse [the process of eating comfort foods and recovering from their negative effects], reducing stress, preventing and treating chronic illness, and prolonging life."[94]

But, I want to encourage you to really take a look at how you feel physically today. Right now, as you read this sentence, *do you feel good*? Are you wishing you could do something about it? You can.

I did. Against my own cynicism, I lost close to a hundred pounds and found a new passion for hiking. It wasn't easy, and keeping it off isn't either. My body is still broken in places from my military and sports careers, but it can handle some footsteps on the trail. Others have taken up other sports, or "shaking and dancing."[95] Whatever the case, we're doing a whole lot of sitting around these days in the 21st century, so the basic cure is to *get the body and blood flowing*. (Or to borrow those quotable words from Michelle Obama: "Let's move!")

I'm just a dude writing a book that you happen to be reading. But remember: you are worth it. And you can do it if you choose to. It's a step towards healing what is broken in you. It stands to reason, then, that you would take the first step towards the person you long to be. When you feel better physically, you will be more apt to find yourself receiving of the Five Ls your loved ones have intricately woven into their lives with you. They care enough for you, and it's time for you to care enough for you, too.

DO YOUR SOUL GOOD

As I mentioned earlier, dealing with something as multifaceted as trauma requires a multi-faceted approach. Human beings are *spiritual* creatures as much as biological, psychological, and social creatures. Read any history of civilization, and some of the distinct characteristics of our species is pondering the depths and meaning of life (philosophy), prayer and meditation (spiritual practice), and developing rituals, beliefs, and narratives about the big picture so we can better organize our lives (religion/theology)—all of which involves symbolic representation (language). Many books on trauma focus on spiritual aspects precisely because they foster genuine healing.

As you've probably already gathered, I'm one of those people who thinks this is meant to be, not an accident of sterile, mindless nature. We were *meant* to be spiritual, *meant* to depend on something greater than ourselves, *meant* to probe the depths of reality, and construct reflections that help us orient ourselves on this brief journey called life.

In our late modern or "post-modern world," this whole orientation has fallen on the rocks. Institutional religion and much of what it offers, at least in the western world, is basically toast. For example, 6,500 people leave Christianity every 24 hours (mostly in the English-speaking world)[96] and 3,500 churches close their doors each year. And it's not without good reason: centuries of crusades, religious wars killing thousands, 9/11 and other religious fundamentalisms, cult movements, televangelist preachers preying on the weak and needy, religious institutions covering up mass child abuse, institutionalized racism and sexism, total rejection of sexual and gender minorities, broken promises about history and infallible books, etc. I've experienced much of this first hand (and much of it is as traumatizing as anything else.)[97] Like many others, I've grown disillusioned with some of the religious systems and ideas that I've become accustomed to.

So, I won't try to justify or promote anything; all kinds of dead wood needs burning in the soul of our country and soul of our world. But I will say this: *our spiritual aspect—our hungers and meditations— are there for good reason, and we must attend to them to be whole.* They are not, as the modern materialist account would have it, a temporary fluke of nature—the product of our desire for an imaginary heavenly father (Freud), a delusionary drug for a discontented people (Marx), a product of society that reinforces the tribe (Durkheim), a temporary survival mechanism we need to shed for human progress, or any of the other reductionistic dismissal. I'm reminded of what Oxford literary critic and novelist C. S. Lewis said:

> If we find ourselves with a desire that nothing in this world can satisfy, the most probable explanation is that we were made for another world.[98]

What if, as human beings get further and further out of survival mode, we become more and more spiritual? (This is what has happened so far.) What if our thirst for a bigger story and a deeper relationship is actually pointing towards something we need, and was part of the plan for this world all along?[99] It's at least something to ponder.

Whatever the case, all of us have our heroes, our sources of inspiration, live according to some philosophy of life, and worship our gods—whether those gods are money, status, sex, power, or a principle, an idea, or a Person. Ultimately, "There's no view from nowhere," as the saying goes. And like others, I find my energy and motivation in the life and teachings of Jesus—who embodied a path forward for life and human flourishing. I began the chapter on leadership with a quote from one of the greatest leaders in all of American history: Ida B. Wells. In December of 1891, she delivered a speech to the American Association of Colored Educators entitled "The Requisites of True Leadership," where she remarked:

> The world has never witnessed a sublime example of love for humanity than that of our blessed Savior whose life on earth was spent in doing good. We cannot hope to equal the infinite love, tenderness and patience with which He taught and served fallen humanity, but we can approximate it. Only in proportion as we do so is our leadership true.[100]

This is the challenge I've come to accept and wrestle with every day. In some ways, my work in writing this book is just as miraculous as my story(ies) of survival: an optimist who struggles with the cynicism of broken people. It seems that no matter what type of service or love you give to these *needy needy* people, they don't accept it, or they push against you. They lie, stab you in the back, ruin your life and others, appreciate nothing, all while you stretch out your arm to them. It doesn't take much to paint all people with this broad brush of hopelessness, and fall into despair. This is "The Way Things Are."[101] How can our tiny efforts really matter, anyway?

I've spent my entire adult life either serving in the military, as a police officer, pastor, military advocate, and now a fresh author trying to spread this great love I've described throughout the book, and I know my limits of carrying others' burdens. I'm aware of this toxic cynicism and its paralyzing effects. But in my walk, it is precisely in those moments that I remember the one who truly loved, beat the odds, and somehow persevered in serving all the dirty, annoying, thankless creatures we call "people." And I remember that I do not carry these burdens alone, and cannot carry the burdens of our whole world anyway.

> Are you tired? Worn out? Burned out on religion? Come to me. Get away with me and you'll recover your life. I'll show you how to take a real rest. Walk with me and work with me—watch how I do it. Learn the unforced rhythms of grace. I won't lay anything heavy or ill-fitting on you. Keep company with me and you'll learn to live freely and lightly. (Matthew 11:28-30, MSG)

In short, my faith has played a crucial role in not only healing and relieving stress, but in inspiring me to Love, Listen, Learn, Lessen, and Lead. I hope you can find a similar source of inspiration and framework of interpretation for life.

CONCLUSION

Most of all, I hope you've found something useful and energizing about this book. I hope you've learned to stop asking "What's wrong with that person?" and start saying, "What happened to that person, and how can I help?" And I hope that you'll come to have hope. Because hope is real, and it's closer than you may realize.

CONCLUDING REFLECTIONS

If you stumbled on this final page and you're on the edge of life itself, I'm here to tell you:

Put the gun down. Push the bottle of pills away. Death is not the only option, and death does not have the last word. You are real. You are unique. You were created for a purpose. Turn away, now, and start looking for love again, because that is what will renew your life. There are people out there who will walk with you. Do what you can to find them. In the meantime, clean house: do good for your body, good for your mind, good for your soul, and good for your relationships, with whatever ounce of strength you have left.

Change begins today.

APPENDIX A:
RELEVANT RESOURCES

There are amazing (and endless) resources out there relating to the themes and goals of this book. But sticking to "my own sphere" and experience, these are just a handful of ones that I thought were worth mentioning.

Books on Compassion and Love in an Evil World
Courtney, Jeremy. *Love Anyway: An Invitation Beyond a World that's Scary as Hell.* Grand Rapids: Zondervan, 2019.
Drietcer, Andrew. *Living Compassion.* Nashville: Upper Room Books, 2017.
Rogers Jr., Frank. *Practicing Compassion.* Nashville: Fresh Air Books, 2015.
McKnight, Scott. *The Jesus Creed.* Brewster: Paraclete Press, 2019.

Relevant Organizations
Culturally Intelligent Training and Consulting LLC
    https://www.culturallyintelligent.com/
Huts for Vets.
    https://hutsforvets.org/
Preemptive Love Coalition.
    https://preemptivelove.org/
Pat Tillman Veteran's Center.
    https://veterans.asu.edu/
The Center for Engaged Compassion.
    http://www.centerforengagedcompassion.com/

NOTES AND REFERENCES

[1] James S. Gordon, *The Transformation: Discovering Wholeness and Healing After Trauma* (New York: HarperOne, 2019), 31.

[2] Office of Mental Health and Suicide Prevention, "2019 National Veteran Suicide Prevention Annual Report" (September 2019). U.S. Department of Veterans Affairs. Available online at: https://www.mentalhealth.va.gov/docs/data-sheets/2019/2019_National_Veteran_Suicide_Prevention_Annual_Report_508.pdf

[3] And no, it's simply and historically untrue that wars like we experience today have always existed or that suicide rates like we experience today have always existed. They have not.

[4] For a similar experience by another author on trauma, note Arielle Schwartz, *The Post-Traumatic Growth Guidebook: Practical Mind-Body Tools to Heal Trauma, Foster Resilience, and Awaken Your Potential* (Eau Claire: PESI Publishing and Media, 2020), xxi.

[5] Just moments before this book went off to the press, I became aware of Schwartz's "6 Rs: Relating, Resourcing, Reprocessing, Repatterning, and Resilience." I obviously find the parallels of this process to the Five Ls fascinating, since they were developed independently and in a different context.

[6] PTSD first entered into the vocabulary of psychiatry and mental health around 1980.

[7] I.e., "concupiscence."

[8] The Greek terms are ἀγάπη (noun) and ἀγαπάω (verb). The three main verbal uses in Koiné are: (1) to have a warm regard for and interest in another, *cherish, have affection for, love;* (2) to have high esteem for or satisfaction with someth., *take pleasure in;* and (3) to practice/express love, *prove one's love.* See William Arndt, Frederick W. Danker, and Walter Bauer, *A Greek-English Lexicon of the New Testament and Other Early Christian Literature*, 3rd ed. (Chicago: University of Chicago Press, 2000), 5-6.

[9] "…insofar as the good of another person is taken, as it were, to be our own good, on account of the union of love, we delight in the good which is done by us for others, especially for friends, as we would in our own good." *Summa Theologica* I-II, question 32. Cf. David Gallagher, "Thomas Aquinas on Self-Love as the Basis for Love of Others," *Acta Philosophica* 8 (1999): 23-44, at 31. Aquinas represents some of the most "classical" of Christian thought. For an introduction to that spiritual and intellectual tradition, see Thomas Oden, *Classic Christianity* (New York: HarperOne, 2009). For a handful of significant, newer innovations to that tradition, see Brian McLaren, *The Great Spiritual Migration: How the World's Largest Religion Is Seeking a Better Way to Be Christian* (New York: Convergent Books, 2017); Sallie McFague, *Collected Readings* (Minneapolis: Fortress Press, 2013); Dorothy Soelle, *Thinking About God* (Eugene: Wipf and Stock, 2016); Jürgen Moltmann, *The Living God and the Fullness of Life* (Minneapolis: Fortress Press, 2015); Marcus Borg, *The Heart of Christianity* (New York: HarperOne, 2003).

[10] Saint Paul's first letter to the Corinthians, as rendered in the CEB.

[11] The classic discussion on these distinctions is C. S. Lewis, *The Four Loves* (New York: Harper Collins, 2017, orig. 1960). One must be careful not to overstate these distinctions, however. See John S. Kloppenborg, "Love In The NT," ed. Katharine Doob Sakenfeld, *The*

New Interpreter's Dictionary of the Bible (Nashville, TN: Abingdon Press, 2006–2009).

[12] The great 20th century intellectual Owen Barfield (colleague of both Tolkien and Lewis), remarked in 1961 that "perhaps the one which fills thoughtful people with the greatest foreboding is the growing general sense of *meaninglessness*. It is this which underlies most of the other threats. How is it that the more able we become to manipulate the world to our advantage, the less we can perceive any meaning in it?" Owen Barfield, *The Rediscovery of Meaning* (Middletown: Wesleyan, 2013, orig. 1977), 13.

[13] Even Jean Baptiste-Say, in contrast to Adam Smith's self-interested individualism, noted that people can and do and should think about how the state of society affects our own individual lives. "…each individual is interested in the general prosperity of all, and that the success of one branch of industry promotes that of all the others. In fact, whatever profession or line of business a man may devote himself to, he is the better paid and the more readily finds employment, in proportion as he sees others thriving equally around him." "A Treatise on Political Economy," cited in Steven G. Medema and Warren J. Samuels, eds., *The History of Economic Thought: A Reader,* 2nd ed. (New York: Routledge, 2013), 260.

[14] A classic and highly influential work on this topic is Friedrich Engels, *The Conditions of the Working Classes in England* (New York: Oxford World Classics,), though short stories like *A Christmas Carol* by Charles Dickens, or "The Little Match Girl" by Hans Christian Andersen are more accessible and vivid portrayals. For an excellent social and political analysis of this problem, see Rudolph Rocker, *Anarcho-Syndicalism: Theory and Practice* (Oakland: AK Press, 2004, orig. 1934).

[15] Jackson Spielvogel, *Western Civilization: A Brief History,* 11th ed. (Boston: Cengage, 2021), 629.

[16] For a concise analysis of some of the problems of our individualist, neoliberal economy, see Jamin Andreas Hübner, "Owning Up to It: How Cooperatives Create the Humane Economy Our World Needs," *Faith and Economics* 76 (2020): 133-208.

[17] "Othering" is a practice typically attributed to colonialism. Lois Tyson, *Critical Theory Today*, 3rd ed. (New York: Routledge, 2015), 401, explains: "The colonizers saw themselves as the embodiment of what a human begin should be, the proper 'self'; native peoples were considered 'other,' different, and therefore inferior to the point of being less than fully human. This practice of judging all who are different as less than fully human is called *othering,* and it divides the world between 'us' (the 'civilized') and 'them' (the 'others,' the 'savages')."

[18] Schwartz, *The Post-Traumatic Growth Guidebook*, 2.

[19] It is no surprise that just before the quote on love in 1 Corinthians 13, the author describes love in these organic, communal terms.

[20] Rogers, *Practicing Compassion*, 16-18.

[21] Not to mention more thorough writings than my own on this subject, such as Frank Rogers Jr., *Practicing Compassion* (Nashville: Fresh Air Books, 2015) and Andrew Drietcer, *Living Compassion* (Nashville: Upper Room Books, 2017).

[22] Rogers, *Practicing Compassion*, 18.

[23] Blaise Pascal, *Pensées* (New York: Penguin Classics, 1995), 13.

[24] Bessel van der Kolk, *The Body Keeps the Score: Brain, Mind, and Body in the Healing of Trauma* (New York: Penguin Books, 2015), 21.

[25] Rogers, *Practicing Compassion*, 18.

[26] George Yancy, *Backlash: What Happens When We Talk Honestly about Racism in America*

(Lanham: Rowman and Littlefield, 2018). If you're skeptical about racism in American history and its effects on the present, also see Ibram X. Kendi, *Stamped from the Beginning: The Definitive History of Racist Ideas in America* (New York: Bold Type Books, 2016) in combination with Henry Louis Gates Jr., *Life Upon These Shores* (New York: Knopf, 2011.

[27] Rogers, *Practicing Compassion*, 18-19.

[28] Rachel Held Evans, "On Forgiveness and Abuse," (August 5, 2014), available online at rachelheldevans.com (accessed October 28, 2020). Perhaps also relevant here, though in a different dimension, is Sarah Schulman, *Conflict Is Not Abuse: Overstating Harm, Community Responsibility, and the Duty of Repair* (Vancouver: Arsenal Pulp Press, 2016).

[29] Gordon, *The Transformation*, 275.

[30] Cf. Schwartz, *The Post Traumatic Growth Handbook*, 194: "forgiveness is an inside job. Your choice to forgive does not let the other person off the hook and does not require that you reconcile or befriend someone that harmed you. However, forgiveness can help you to have compassion for them despite their hurtful actions. Part of this process involves having empathy for their circumstances…in finding forgiveness, you let go of the need to retaliate or punish the person who hurt you."

[31] Richard Rohr, "Transforming Pain." The Center for Action and Contemplation (October 17, 2018). Available online at: https://cac.org/transforming-pain-2018-10-17/

[32] John 15:13 (CEB).

[33] This creates a special kind of trauma—PITS (Perpetration Induced Traumatic Stress). See Mark Charles and Soong-Chan Rah, *Unsettling Truths* (Downers Grove: InterVarsity, 2019), 174-76 and Rachel McNair, *Perpetration-Induced Traumatic Stress: The Psychological Consequences of Killing* (Lincoln: iUniverse, 2005).

[34] Paul Bloom, *Against Empathy: The Case for Rational Compassion* (New York: Ecco, 2016).

[35] See the many lectures and writings of Jordan Peterson.

[36] Kristin Kobes DuMez, *Jesus and John Wayne: How White Evangelicals Corrupted a Faith and Divided a Nation* (New York: Liveright, 2020). Cf. the film *Won't You Be My Neighbor?* (2018).

[37] See Chris Hedges, interview with Laura Flanders, "GRITtv: Chris Hedges: Demonizing Empathy," (May 12, 2011, available online at: https://youtu.be/6w4hpeCGTG0 (accessed October 28, 2020); Perry L. Glanzer, "The Demise of Gentleness," *Christian Scholars Review* blog (October 30, 2020), available online at: https://christianscholars.com/the-demise-of-gentleness.

[38] This problem is embodied in nationalistic politics, where loving refugees (giving them food and water and making sure, say, kids at the southern border don't starve to death) is considered traitorous.

[39] Zurich, "Decline in Human Empathy Creates Global Risks in the 'Age of Anger'," (April 9, 2019), available online at: https://www.zurich.com/en/knowledge/topics/global-risks/decline-human-empathy-creates-global-risks-age-of-anger

[40] See David Bentley Hart, *Atheist Delusions* (New Haven: Yale University Press, 2009), 104-109: "We live now in the wake of the most monstrously violent century in human history, during which the secular order (on both the political right and the political left), freed from the authority of religion, showed itself willing to kill on an unprecedented scale and with an ease of conscience worse than merely depraved. If ever an age deserved to be thought an age of darkness, it is surely ours… Christian society certainly never fully purged itself of cruelty or violence; but it also never incubated evils comparable in ambition, range, systematic precision, or mercilessness to death camps, gulags, forced famines, or the extravagant brutality of modern warfare."

[41] Schwartz, *The Post Traumatic Growth Handbook,* 80.

[42] Liz Ford, "Nine out of 10 people found to be biased against women," *The Guardian* (March 5, 2020).

[43] Christina Zhao, "Amid Tributes, Sean Connery's Views on Slapping Women Have Been Largely Overlooked," *Newsweek* (October 31, 2020).

[44] Statistics from federal websites and Statista.com show that 97% of veteran suicides are male when 91% of the U.S. military is male. According to the American Foundation for Suicide Prevention (https://afsp.org/suicide-statistics/), men die by suicide 3.53x more often than women.

[45] See Joshua Klugman, "Do 40% of police families experience domestic violence?" (July 20, 2020). Available online at https://sites.temple.edu/klugman/2020/07/20/do-40-of-police-families-experience-domestic-violence/. The primary sources for these statistics are: L. B. Johnson, "On the front lines: Police stress and family well-being. Hearing before the Select Committee on Children, Youth, and Families House of Representatives: 102 Congress First Session," (May 20, 1991): 32-48; Washington DC: US Government Printing Office and P.H. Neidig, H.E. Russell, A. F. Seng, "Interspousal aggression in law enforcement families: A preliminary investigation," *Police Studies* 15:1 (1992): 30-38.

[46] Gordon, *The Transformation,* 82.

[47] Stephen Mitchel, trans., *Tao Te Ching: A New English Version* (New York: Perennial Classics, 2006), no. 76.

[48] Augustine, *On Christian Teaching,* trans. R. P. H. Green (New York: Oxford University Press, 1997), I.28.29.

[49] Cornel West, *Black Prophetic Fire* (Boston: Beacon Press, 2014), 66.

[50] Ibram X. Kendi, *How to Be An Antiracist* (New York: New World, 2019), 46-47, critiques the use of "microaggressions" because "A persistent daily low hum of racist abuse is not minor…What other people call racial microaggressions I call racist abuse." I use it here because of its contemporary currency amongst sociologists and general validity, and do not in any way suggest that microaggressions are a "minor" issue, especially in their cumulative effect.

[51] See for example, Kendi's *How to be AntiRacist* in conjunction with Derald Wing Sue and Lisa Spanierman, *Microaggressions in Everyday Life,* 2nd ed. (New York: Wiley, 2020).

[52] Elaine Bellezza, "Hildegard of Bingen, Warrior of Light," *Gnosis* 21 (Fall 1991). This quote is misattributed to Hildegarde almost everywhere it is found on the internet.

[53] Schwartz, *The Post Traumatic Growth Guidebook,* 31.

[54] Cf. Schwartz, *The Post Traumatic Growth Guidebook,* 44: "Identifying positive moments in addition to your challenges will help you tap into existing strengths." A key work on this subject of constructing one's own identity in relationships is Kenneth Gergen, *An Invitation Social Construction* (London: SAGE, 2015). Narrative therapy focuses on these scripts and stories and how the people in our lives create them and, ultimately, define who we are.

[55] This is no joke. First century Palestinians suffered generational trauma from war, displacement, religious persecution, etc. that stretches back centuries to the beginning of the Second-Temple period (about 586 BCE) all the way into the colonization of Rome. There is now a small library of books that focus on the intersection between trauma and early Jewish and Christian communities.

[56] Important introductory books on the person of Jesus by contemporary scholars include Marcus Borg, *Meeting Jesus Again for the First Time* (New York: HarperOne, 2009); John Dominic Crossan, *Jesus: A Revolutionary Biography* (New York: HarperOne, 2009); N. T.

Wright, *Simply Jesus: A New Vision of Who He Was, What He Did, and Why He Matters* (New York: HarperOne, 2011). See also "The Chosen" video series (https://studios.vidangel.com/the-chosen).

[57] Cf. James Dunn, *Jesus Remembered* (Christianity in the Making Volume 1) (Grand Rapids: Eerdmans, 2003); *idem., Jesus According to the New Testament* (Grand Rapids: Eerdmans, 2019); Craig Keener, *Christobiography: Memory, History, and the Reliability of the Gospels* (Grand Rapids: Eerdmans, 2019); Richard Bauckham, "Gospel Narratives and the Psychology of Eyewitness Memory" in *Christian and the Created Order: Perspectives from Theology, Philosophy, and Science*, ed. Andrew Torrance and Thomas McCall (Grand Rapids: Zondervan, 2018).

[58] Isaiah 61:1, cited by Jesus in Luke 4:18.

[59] van der Kolk, *The Body Keeps the Score*, 70.

[60] NYU Langone Health / NYU School of Medicine. "Artificial intelligence can diagnose PTSD by analyzing voices: Study tests potential telemedicine approach." *ScienceDaily* (22 April 2019). Available at www.sciencedaily.com/releases/2019/04/190422082232.htm.

[61] See the 2016 DoD SAPR Annual Report. Available at https://www.rand.org/nsrd/projects/rmws/publications.html and https://www.sapr.mil/sites/default/files/_DoD_Annual_Report_on_Sexual_Harassment_and_Violence_APY18-19.pdf

[62] Robert Wilken, *The Spirit of Early Christian Thought* (New Haven: Yale University Press, 2005), 172, 183.

[63] Cf. the very brief summary of Polyvagal Theory and neurological hierarchy in Schwartz, *The Post Traumatic Growth Handbook*, 15ff.

[64] Mental Health Systems, "Parasympathetic Nervous System and Trauma," MHS (March 2, 2020). Available online at: https://www.mhs-dbt.com/blog/parasympathetic-nervous-system-and-trauma/

[65] Van der Kolk, *The Body Keeps the Score*, 56, 53.

[66] Van der Kolk, *The Body Keeps the Score*, 63-64. EMDR (Eye-Movement and Desensitization Reprocessing) is a new and promising therapy for those with PTSD. See https://www.emdr.com/what-is-emdr/

[67] Cf. van der Kolk, *The Body Keeps the Score*, 70.

[68] Cf. Schwartz, *The Post Traumatic Growth Guidebook*, 34, which frames this problem as one of "three myths." The other two are "time heals all wounds" and "the belief that 'you should be over this by now'."

[69] Van der Kolk, *The Body Keeps the Score*, 25: "If you do something to a patient that you would not do to your friends or children, consider whether you are unwittingly replicating a trauma from this patient's past."

[70] Van der Kolk, *The Body Keeps the Score*, 127.

[71] Chris Hedges, *What Every Person Needs to Know About War* (New York: Free Press, 2003).

[72] Michael White, *Maps of Narrative Practice* (New York: Norton & Norton, 2007), 103.

[73] Van der Kolk, *The Body Keeps the Score*, 64.

[74] Van der Kolk, *The Body Keeps the Score*, 101.

[75] Van der Kolk, *The Body Keeps the Score*, 192.

[76] If you feel your life is in danger as the result of such encouragement, then this is a bit different. I'm not suggesting that you should risk or endure violence. In fact, you never should; if your life is threatened in any situation with a partner, it may be time to draw firmer boundaries and/or bail the relationship.

---

[77] Schwartz, *The Post Traumatic Growth Handbook,* 72: "The practice of grounding, which arises from somatic or body=based psychotherapy, can help you reconnect to yourself — your center. Grounding refers to your ability to feel yourself here and now. Through sensory awareness, you bring your attention to your body. What do you see, hear, smell, taste, and touch? You can amplify your sensory experience in the outdoors by slowly sensing the texture of a tough rock with your finger tips or smelling the fresh pine sap in the bark of a tree. Grounding also emphasizes bringing awareness to your legs and feet by sensing your connection to earth."

[78] Henry David Thoreau, cited in Henry S. Butler, *Moments of Wilderness: Exploring Nature in the Search for Meaning* (Indianapolis: Dog Ear Publishing, 2017), 226.

[79] Cited in Charles Roy, ed., *Albert Schweitzer: An Anthology* (Boston: Beacon Press, 1947), 248.

[80] Those interested in the connections between the sciences, philosophy, and amazing features of nature, see Ursula Goodenough, *The Sacred Depths of Nature* (New York: Oxford University Press, 1998); Benjamin Wiker and Jonathan Witt, *A Meaningful World: How the Arts and Sciences Reveal the Genius of Nature* (Downers Grove: IVP Academic, 2006); Guillermo Gonzalez and Jay Richards, *The Privileged Planet* (Washington D. C.: Regnery, 2020). For excellent works specifically addressing the relationship between science and religion, see Philip Clayton, *Science and Religion: The Basics* (New York: Routledge, 2018) and Philip Clayton, *God and Gravity,* ed. Bradford McCall (Eugene: Cascade, 2018).

[81] Gordon, *The Transformation,* 209.

[82] Gordon, *The Transformation,* 214.

[83] Schwartz, *The Post Traumatic Growth Handbook,* 73.

[84] "Klick" is military slang for kilometer.

[85] This should not be confused with the similar phenomenon of scapegoating in anthropology (the tendency of the group to pin responsibility on a particular person in order to maintain social order and alleviate the group's own guilt). René Girard explored this theme perhaps more deeply than anyone else, at least when trying to understand the emergence of religious sacrifice.

[86] Aldo Leopold, "Thinking Like a Mountain," *EPA Journal* 14:1 (May 1988): 2.

[87] Alan Kreider, *The Patient Ferment of the Early Church: The Improbable Rise of Christianity in the Roman Empire* (Grand Rapids: Baker Academic, 2016).

[88] The cross in Christianity also resembles an icon of transformative love. Crucifixion — perhaps the most traumatic event we could think of — was reserved for revolutionaries and rebels in the Roman empire. So the cross of crucifixion was a symbol of death, torture, and punishment meant to instill fear into the lives of any agitator. But, in the Hebrew tradition of turning "swords into ploughshares," Jesus transformed the evil cross into something good and redemptive — into a symbol of love itself. It's my conviction that we are to do the same today: transform and redeem everything bad in this world into something good and flourishing.

[89] Schwartz, *The Post-Traumatic Guidebook,* 6-7.

[90] Schwartz, *The Post-Traumatic Guidebook,* 7.

[91] Gordon, *The Transformation,* 56-57.

[92] Cf. Schwartz, *The Post Traumatic Growth Guidebook,* 6: "…resilience is grounded in realistic optimism, which involves maintaining a positive outlook on life while simultaneously acknowledging the challenges that will occur along the way."

[93] Gordon, *The Transformation,* 217.

[94] Gordon, *The Transformation,* 142. Cf. Schwartz, *The Post Traumatic Growth Handbook,* 87: "Exercise in particular provides you with a natural chemical boost that lifts mood by increasing endorphins, serotonin, and norepinephrine. You can also increase resilience by maintaining a healthy digestive system."

[95] Gordon, *The Transformation,* 72.

[96] See the first chapter of Jamin Andreas Hübner, *Deconstructing Evangelicalism: A Letter to a Friend and a Professor's Guide to Escaping Religious Fundamentalism* (Rapid City: Hills Publishing Group, 2020).

[97] See Teresa Pasquale, *Sacred Wounds: A Path to Healing from Spiritual Trauma* (Danvers: Chalice Press, 2015); Connie Baker, *Traumatized by Religious Abuse: Courage, Hope and Freedom for Survivors* (Eugene: Luminare Press, 2019).

[98] C. S. Lewis, *Mere Christianity* (New York: HarperOne, 2015, orig 1952).

[99] See John Haught, *The New Cosmic Story: Inside Our Awakening Universe* (New Haven: Yale University, 2017).

[100] Ida B. Wells, "The Requisites of True Leadership" in *The Light of Truth: Writings of an Anti-Lynching Crusader,* ed. Henry Louis Gates Jr. and Mia Bay (New York: Penguin Classics, 2014), 41.

[101] See Jeremy Courtney, *Love Anyway* (Grand Rapids: Zondervan, 2019).

CPSIA information can be obtained
at www.ICGtesting.com
Printed in the USA
FSHW010504060821
83872FS